ALLERGY

WHICH ALLERGENS?

A Service from Pharmacia AB

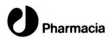 Pharmacia

The manuscript is a product of the combined efforts of: Marie Aginder, Marie-Louise Andrae, Hans Arrendal, Sten Dreborg, David Fisher, Janet Hedenström, Catharina Hemström, Margaret Knipe, Jüri Kurvits, Sig-Britt Nilsson, Wenche Rolfsen, Hans Schröder, Ann-Catarine Westerlund and Lars Yman.

A list of Photographers

OSF Picture Library Oxford England
Photographer/Oxford Scientific Films
Prosopis juliflora t 20.

Photographer Alan Mitchell
Carya pecan t 22, Fraxinus americana t 15,
Pinus strobus t 16, Populus deltoides t 14.

Med. Fact Ohio USA
Juglans californica t 10, Atriplex lentiformis w 15,
Ambrosia psilostachya w 2.

Jörgen Carlsson, Uppsala Sweden
Cat e 1.

Gunnar Carlin, Uppsala Sweden
Alnus incana t 2, Ambrosia trifida w 3,
Poa pratensis g 8, Bromus inermis g 11.

Bildgruppen, Helsingborg Sweden
Photographer Harry Mann.
Mould m 1, m 2, m 4, m 6

Biologiska bildbyrån, Enebyberg Sweden
Photographer Henrik Nordström.
Rumex acetotella w 18, Cryptomeria japonica t 17,
Kochia scoparia w 17.

Johan Holm, Stockholm Sweden
Apis mellifera i 1, Vespula i 3, Hazelnut f 17,
Crab f 23, Egg f 1, Fish Cod f 3, A glass of milk f 2,
Pea f 12, Salix caprea t 12, Artemisia absinthium w 5,
Dactylis glomerata g 3, Avena sativa g 14,
Authoranthum odoratum g 1, Secale cereale g 12,
Triticum sativum g 15, Phragmites communis g 7.

IBL Ljungbyhed, Sweden
Meteorologi, fog m 2 Å. Lindau
Urtica dioica w 20 Å. Lindau
Alopecurus pratensis g 16 K.B.

Bernt Johansson, Uppsala Sweden
Cow e 4, Horse e 3, Guinea pig e 6,
Chrysanthemum leucanthemum w 7.

André Maslemikov, Alunda Sweden
Acer negundo t 1.

Naturfotograferna, Österbybruk Sweden
Blatella germanica i 6, Peter Hanneberg,
Garlic f 47, Onion f 48, Bo Brännhage,
Fagus grandifolia American t 5, Åke W Engman,
Juniperus t 6, Tore Hagman, Cupressus t 23,
Björn-Eyvind Swahn.

Photographer Fagg, Australia
Acacia longifolia t 19, Eucalyptus t 18.

Photographer N Cnops, Belgium
Salsola kali w 11, Chenopodium album w 10,
Solidago virgaurea w 12, Artemisia vulgaris w 6,
Lolium perenne g 5, Phleum pratense g 6.

Crown copyright England
Mite d 1.

Statens Bakteriologiska Laboratorium, Solna Sweden
Egg Schistosoma mansoni p 3,
Cercarie Schistosoma mansoni p 3.

Monica Svensson, Uppsala Sweden
Betula verrucosa t 3

Hasse Schröder, Uppsala Sweden
Olea europaea t 9, Betula verrucosa t 3,
Corylus avellana t 4, Quercus alba t 7,
Platanus acerifolia t 11, Ulmus americana t 8,
Plantago lanceolata w 9, Festuca elatior g 4
Cynodon dactylon g 2 and the Cover-picture.

Mia Schröder, Uppsala Sweden
Dog e 2.

Allergon AB, Välinge Sweden
Amaranthus retroflexus w 14, Holcus lanatus g 13

Atom, Spain
Parietaria officialis w 19, Parietaria judaica w 21

Ardea, London England
Xanthium Spp w 13, JLM
Iva Spp w 16, ROG, Melaleuca spp t 21, DB

01-548
ISBN 91-970475-5-4

Printed in Sweden by Västra Aros, Västerås, 1985

Contents

Introduction

Pioneers in IgE testing

It is now over a decade since the first laboratory test for the determination of total IgE in serum was introduced by Pharmacia.

Since then there have been thousands of articles describing the use of total IgE and specific IgE determinations in establishing a better understanding of the allergic response both in research and clinical practice. During this time reagents from Pharmacia (Phadebas IgE PRIST® and Phadebas RAST®) have been used as the reference on which many scientific and clinical studies have been based.

Pharmacia has placed great emphasis on the commitment to research in allergy and has published hundreds of scientific articles. About 15% of the total turnover is invested in basic research and development. Together with our colleagues in allergy research throughout the world, many new and exciting projects are underway which guarantee Pharmacia's continued pioneering endeavors in the field of immunology.

It is this commitment to a better understanding of the allergic response and the production of high quality reagents that has significantly contributed to the increased knowledge of this complex immunological disturbance.

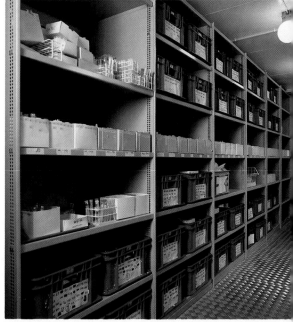

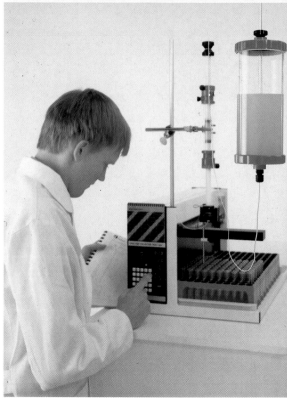

Pharmacia – The allergy company

In the immunotherapy field, the Allergy and Diagnostic Division within the Health Care Group of Pharmacia has been able to draw upon the considerable experience and expertise of both the Fine Chemicals Division in separation technology and the Pharmaceuticals Division in pharmaceutical production and quality control to develop advanced immunotherapy products. This latter work has been carried out in co-operation with Nyegaard & Co in Norway.

Quality products for optimal patient management

The integration of products for diagnosis and immunotherapy using common raw material sources and the same stringent quality control procedures is the security you receive when using Pharmacia's Phadebas RAST®/Phadezym RAST® and Pharmalgen® allergen preparations*.
Many have tried to make reagents for the measurement of allergen specific IgE antibodies, few have succeeded, and none, apart from Pharmacia, have documented the reliability of a wide panel in routine clinical use so thoroughly. The sensitivity and specificity of the Phadebas RAST®/Phadezym RAST® is the result of the combination of high quality of radioactively-labelled or enzyme-labelled antihuman IgE and unique solid phase bound allergens (1,2). Standardization and continuous search for improvements are keys to efficacy.

* The range of *in vivo* products is necessarily smaller due to the additional quality control procedures required.

Quality demands quality control

The products can only be as good as the raw materials they employ. Pharmacia's raw materials are supplied by Allergon AB, the world's leading producer of allergenic raw material and a subsidiary of Pharmacia in southern Sweden. Allergon Inc. in the USA collects pollen from plants which do not grow in Europe. Many species must be cultivated for maximal purity. Each allergen requires its own collection routine to obtain the highest allergenic content.
For example, the pollen with the highest allergenic content may be present for only few hours in some plants. The timing for the collection is therefore critical.
Pollens are analyzed for identity and purity by microscopical and immunochemical tests.
Allergens such as moulds and mites are cultivated on allergen-free synthetic media carefully chosen to suit the special characteristics of the species. Precise cultivation criteria such as temperature, pH and culture age have been developed.

Introduction

Epithelial allergens and other proteins of animal origin require special consideration. Pharmacia has chosen the raw materials after studying the different breeds to ascertain the allergenic content as well as clinical sensitivity of allergic patients to the various breeds. Different preparations such as serum, saliva, dander and 'skin-scrapings' have also been examined to find the best composition for coupling to the allergen discs.

The foods are fresh unless special reasons demand the use of processed material. Much effort has been put into controlling their clinical relevance.

Upon arrival all source materials are subject to analysis for specificity and potency according to strict specifications. The analytical tools include methods like the RAST inhibition (3, 4) CIE/CRIE (5, 6). CEIE (crossed enzyme immuno-electrophoresis) (7) and immunoprint techniques for direct identification of allergen and antibody patterns (8, 9, 10).

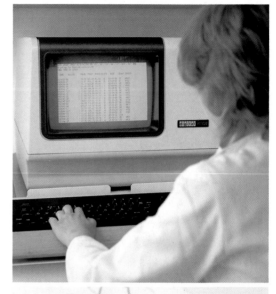

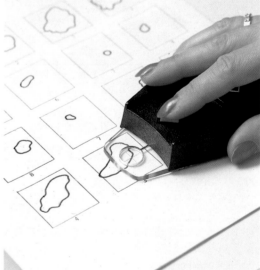

Documented patient sera for testing

An important aspect in product development and quality control is the availability of well characterized allergic serum samples. Pharmacia has a "library" in excess of 13 000 serum samples and is continuously adding samples according to strict selection criteria including complete case history, *in vitro* and *in vivo* tests.

Pharmacia's reliability is well-documented

The clinical documentation supporting these products and referred to throughout these pages is part of the assurance provided when using diagnostic and therapeutic products from Pharmacia.

Using Phadebas RAST®/Phadezym RAST® in conjunction with a careful case history and, where appropriate, skin and provocation tests leads to accurate diagnosis and therefore better discrimination in the treatment choice.

References

1. *de Filippi I., Yman L. and Schröder H.*
   Clinical accuracy updated version of the Phadebas RAST® test.
   Ann Allergy 46 (1981) p. 249.

2. *Schröder H. and Kober A.*
   New developments in specific antibody measurement – Phadezym RAST® correlation between EIA and RIA (Phadebas RAST®).
   Allergologia et Immunopathologia suppl. 9 (1981) p. 46–50.

3. *Yman L., Ponterius G. and Brandt R.*
   RAST-based allergen assay methods.
   Devel biol Standard 29 (Karger Basel, 1975) p. 151–165.

4. *Schröder H. and Yman L.*
   Standardization of the RAST inhibition assay. Allergy 35 (1980) p. 234–236.

5. *Aukrust L.*
   Crossed radioimmunoelectrophoretic studies of distinct allergens in two extracts of Cladosporium herbarum.
   Int Arch Allergy appl Immunol 58 (1979) p. 375–390.

6. *Axelsen N. H.*
   A manual of quantitative immuno-electrophoresis. Methods and applications.
   Scand J Immunol 2 Suppl. 1 (1973).

7. *Andrae M-L., Schröder H. and Yman L.*
   Identification and characterization of allergens by a new crossed enzyme immunoelectrophoretic technique (CEIE) using the Phadezym RAST® tracer.
   J Clin All Clin Immunol 69 (1982) p. 75.

8. *Yman L., Blomberg F. and Schröder H.*
   Characterization of dog and cat allergens. Direct specific detection of electrophoretically separated allergens by means of IgE antibodies and enzyme-labelled anti-IgE.
   In: Adv Allergy Immunol Eds.: A Oehling et al. Perganon press, Oxford, New York (1980) p. 513–519.

9. *Schröder H., Blomberg F. and Yman L.*
   Enzyme immunoassays (EIA) for quantitative and qualitative analysis of allergen extracts.
   In: Adv Allergy Immunol Eds.: A Oehling et al. Perganon press, Oxford, New York (1980) p. 513–519.

10. *Bengtsson A., Rolfsen W. and Einarsson R.*
    A nitrocellulose immunoprint technique for detection of allergic components in allergen preparations and source materials.
    J Allergy Clin Immun Supp 73 (1984) p. 190.

Pollens

Pollens of a rich variety of the plant species are recognized as major causes of allergic manifestations in human beings. The plants of major importance in pollen allergy are mainly those relying on the wind as the carrier.

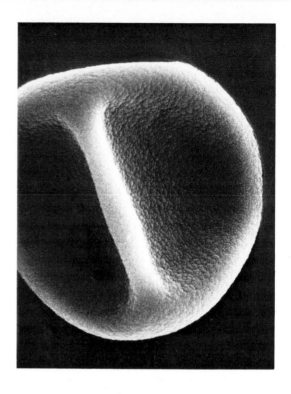

These plants produce large amounts of pollens in order to increase the probability that the grain will reach the pistil of a female flower of the same species. They often shed their light, easily air-borne pollen during a short period ranging from a few hours to few days. Some species develop new flowers continuously thus prolonging the period of time during which pollen can be found in the air. Most of the allergenic plants of the different climate zones of one part of the world are found also in other parts with similar conditions having been spread by natural routes or introduced by man. New varieties or even species showing new shapes of leaves, flowers may have appeared in different regions as a result of evolution, but the allergenic properties do not seem to be influenced by such variation to such a degree that they are recognized by the allergic patient.

Related pollens contain related allergens and the closer they are related the stronger is the immunological cross-reactivity. An allergic patient moving from one area to another may suffer an allergic reaction which due to the cross-reactivity between the pollen allergens of related species.

Knowledge of systematic botany and the geographical distribution of common plants combined with clinical and immunological observations permits selection of adequate allergen panels for diagnosis and therapy.

The Phadebas RAST®/Phadezym RAST® panel covers the world's major allergenic pollens from grasses, trees and weeds found in temperate and tropical regions of both hemispheres. We have grouped the allergens according to their taxonomical relationship. The diagrams will help you find the allergen. We have followed the classification of the late Professor J.A. Nannfelt, Uppsala, Sweden.

I

Graminae*, though not the largest, is certainly the most economically important plant family. Man's dependence on grass probably goes back 8 000 to 10 000 years ago to southwest Asia and the Middle East. Species of *Triticum* and *Hordeum* (wheat and barley) were cultivated. Gradually strains which were best suited to cultivation, such as *Secale cereale* and *Avena sativa* were developed. The second important step was the domestication of animals and the need for grazing lands. Actual storing of hay for fodder dates back to the Romans. In the 12th century, pastures were first sown with rye.

Consisting of roughly 9 000 species, the grasses may cover 20 % of the world's surface. Moreover, several grasses are expanding their territory with man's help through deforestation and import-export activities. Numerous important cereals and forage plants are found within this family, as well as grass mixtures for lawns. The geographical information indicated in the text is approximate for the species, while indicating the genus.

In Europe, inhalation of grass pollens is the predominant cause of hay fever and related hypersensitivity reactions. In northern temperate climates, the peak pollination period extends from May to July. However, in tropical and subtropical regions, the climate permits two or more grass-pollinating seasons annually which may extend from March to November.

The flowers open for only a few hours to permit pollination. The pollen itself is viable for less than 1 day, the shortest-lived of all flowering pollen plants. The flowering seasons indicated in the text are approximate and based on agricultural, horticultural and botanical source material.

All of the Phadebas RAST®/Phadezym RAST® grass pollen allergen discs are produced by coupling an allergen extract of a pure preparation of grass pollen to activated paper discs.

* Syn. *Poainae*

Botanical relations

This schema is one of many possible organizations of grasses. Taxonomy and nomenclature have been debated since the time of Aristotle and there appears to be no end in sight.

Grasses

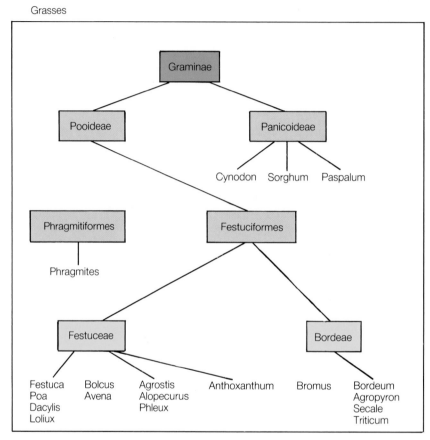

The genera followed by the species are listed alphabetically in the text. All the grasses belong to a single family of about 9 000 species. The family can be divided into two subfamilies, the *Pooideae* and the *Panicoideae*. The subfamily *Pooideae* contains two groups, the *Phragmitiformes* and the *Festuciformes*. The group, *Festuciformes*, can be further divided into a number of tribes that include *Festuceae* and *Nordeae*, which contain most of the widespread grasses. The distribution for *Festuceae* is grouped in the text as seen here in the diagram.

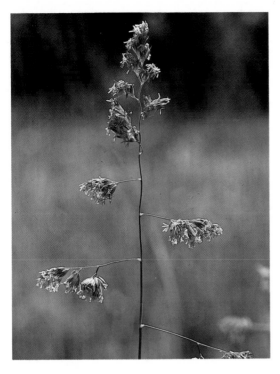

Cocksfoot is a valuable forage grass and is also found in open ground, meadows and moist places. It is one of the best grasses for cultivating in shady areas.

It is widespread in Europe and North America and is found in other parts of the world, e.g. in Japan, where it is a major pollen source and in Great Britain, France and Germany.

In North America it flowers from April/May to August and in Europe from June to September. It begins growing early in the spring and has strong re-growth after grazing.

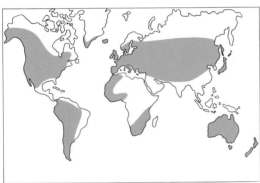

Cocksfoot allergens seems to cross-react with those of Timothy, g6 (72). In a number of studies (33, 50, 51) a higher incidence of hypersensitivity has been found to Cocksfoot than to other grass species.

Phadebas RAST®/Phadezym RAST® allergen g3 is acknowledged to be highly sensitive and specific (80).

References: 33, 50, 51, 72, 80

Further reading: 2, 7, 10, 39, 54, 55, 56, 59, 61 , 63, 64, 65, 66, 68, 69, 70, 95

Meadow fescue is an important
member of the "lawn" family
as it has a very fine texture. It is
a temperate climate grass,
cultivated for forage and meadow.
It is also cultivated as a soil-
conserving plant.

Meadow fescue can be found
throughout most of Europe.
It has also been introduced and
cultivated in North America.
Meadow fescue flowers in early
summer.

Naturally, a high degree of cross-
reactivity to other species of the
same genus is found. Cross-
reactivity can also be expected
with Timothy (g6), Cocksfoot (g3),
Meadow grass (g8) as well as with
Rye-grass (g5) and Velvet grass
(g13) (72).

Phadebas RAST®/Phadezym
RAST® allergen g4 is
acknowledged to be highly
sensitive and specific (71).

References: 71, 72

Further reading: 2, 7, 10, 33, 51, 54,
61, 65

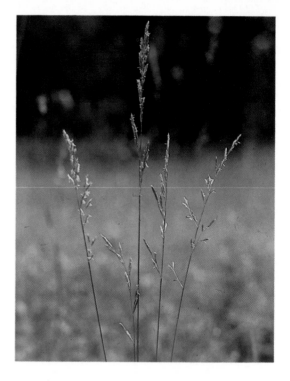

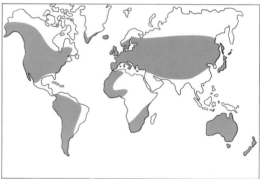

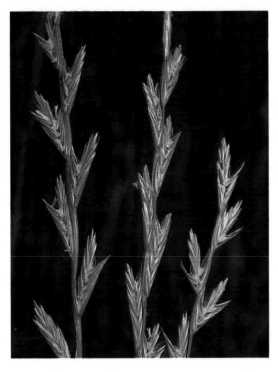

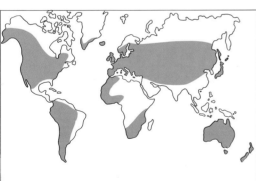

Rye-grass is blended in lawn seed mixtures and is widely cultivated in temperate leys in Europe for grazing, hay and ensilage. It was the first meadow grass cultivated in Europe, and is considered the most important forage grass there.

It is native to Europe and was introduced in North and South America as well as temperate Asia and Australia.

Rye-grass may flower almost all summer.

High cross-reactivity is shown to other species within the genus *Lolium* but it is moderate with Velvet grass (g13), Timothy (g6), Meadow grass (g8) and Cocksfoot (g3) (72).

Phadebas RAST®/Phadezym RAST® allergen g5 is acknowledged to be highly sensitive and specific (2, 33, 61).

References: 2, 33, 61, 72

Further reading: 4, 7, 31, 50, 51, 65, 69, 84, 85, 91, 93, 95, 252

Meadow grass is a tuft-forming perennial often cultivated for forage and commonly found in lawns. It is probably the most important introduced grass in North America.

Meadow grass is native to the Old World and Eurasia. Most of the 200 species of the genus *Poa* are distributed in the cold and temperate regions of the world. It is a major pollen-producer throughout Canada, the northeastern United States and in European countries such as France and Belgium.

Meadow grass flowers in early or midsummer and is a cool-season grass.

Meadow grass is a very complex species having several recognized forms highly cross-reactive to each other (72).

Phadebas RAST®/Phadezym RAST® allergen g8 is acknowledged to be highly sensitive and specific (2, 33, 51).

References: 2, 33, 51, 72

Further reading: 4, 10, 61

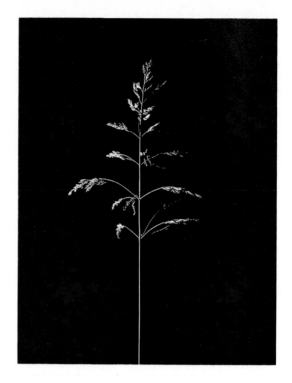

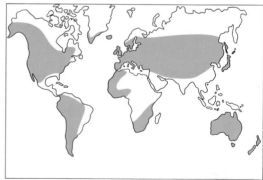

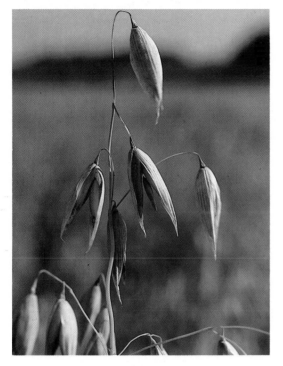

Wild oats may be the origin of this cultivated form, now used for human and animal food. Oats have been cultivated since classical times in cooler climates. The plant has given rise to such colloquial expressions as 'off one's oats', 'feel one's oats' and 'sow one's wild oats'.

The major growing areas are the USA, southern Canada, the USSR and Europe particularly around the Mediterranean.

Oat flowers in midsummer.

In RAST-inhibition studies, a low degree of cross-reactivity to other grass pollens has been indicated (147).

References: 147

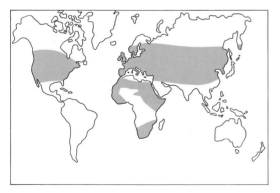

I:7

Velvet grass is a perennial grass, common in open woods, fields and in waste areas. The name velvet grass comes from the appearance its pale purple flower heads make when growing amassed in an open field. In many countries *H. lanatus* is considered a weed and only of minor importance for grazing.

Velvet grass is common in most of Europe, though it is absent in the northernmost regions. It is also found in temperate Asia. It was introduced in North America where it is occasionally cultivated as meadow.

Velvet grass flowers in late summer.

Cross-reactivity can be expected to other member of the *Holcus* genus as well as to other members of the tribe (72).

Phadebas RAST®/Phadezym RAST® allergen g13 is acknowledged to be highly sensitive and specific (146).

References: 72, 146

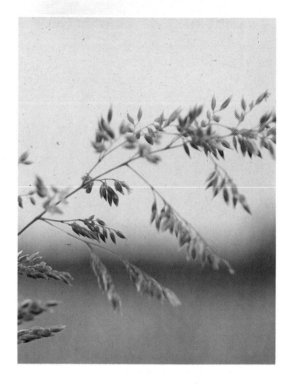

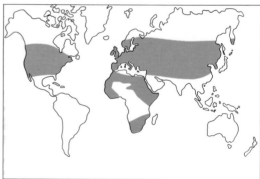

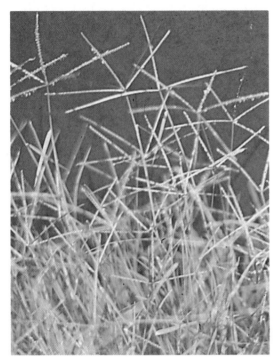

Redtop is often cultivated as a member of the "lawn" family. It is one of the best wetland tame grasses. No other grass can adapt to so wide range of soils and climatic conditions.

Redtop is a native of the Old World, found in Europe, Asia and West Africa. It was first cultivated in the US in the 1800's and ranges from Canada to the Gulf Coast. It was also introduced in Australia, New Zealand and South Africa.

Redtop flowers in mid- and late summer.

Redtop is highly cross-reactive to Timothy (g6), Meadow grass (g8), Cocksfoot (g3) and Rye-grass (g5) (72).

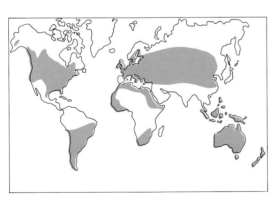

Phadebas RAST®/Phadezym RAST® allergen g9 is acknowledged to be highly sensitive and specific (80).

References: 72, 80

Meadow foxtail is a sought-after forage grass valuable because it is both succulent and hardy. It is especially suited to swampy, overflow lands. It is traditionally included in mixed grass pollen extracts for skin testing.

Meadow foxtail is native to Europe and Asia and is cultivated for forage in Australia, New Zealand and North America though there not considered to be a major pollen-producer.

It is one of the first grasses to begin growth in the spring and in mild climates it can grow throughout the winter season. In colder climates it blooms from April to July. The stamens are first yellow then become orange.

A high degree of cross-reactivity can be expected between Meadow foxtail and Cocksfoot (g3), Meadow fescue (g4), Rye-grass (g5), Timothy (g6) and Meadow grass (g8) (72).

References: 72

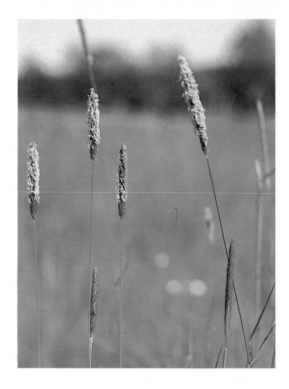

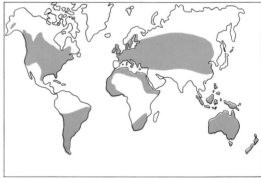

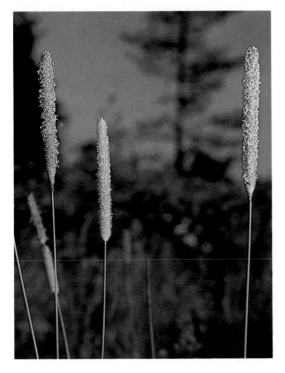

Timothy is one of the primary sources of animal fodder. It grows also in meadows and grasslands, often along roadsides and waste places. It is one of the world's most common grasses and grows best in cooler, humid climates.

Timothy is native and common in most of Europe, North Africa and northern Asia. It has been introduced in North and South America, South Africa and Australia.

Phelum pratense flowers in the summer in Europe and North America.

Timothy seems highly cross-reactive to other species of the genus *Phleum* as well as moderately with species of other genera such as Meadow fescue (g4), Velvet grass (g13), Rye-grass (g5), Meadow grass (g8) and Cocksfoot (g3) (72).

Phadebas RAST®/Phadezym RAST® allergen g6 is acknowledged to be highly sensitive and specific (2, 51, 97, 98, 101, 102, 103).

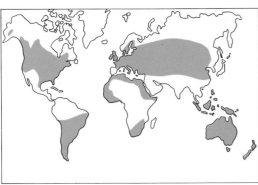

References: 2, 51, 72, 97, 98, 101, 102, 103

Further reading: 4, 10, 39, 54, 61, 62, 65, 66, 69, 91, 95, 104, 105, 106, 107, 108, 109, 113, 1 16, 118, 119, 120, 121, 123, 128, 129, 132, 134, 201

Sweet vernal grass is a perennial grass with a sweet scent of coumarin similar to that of new-mown hay. When eaten it has a taste similar to a caramel though the grass is unpalatable for livestock. It is a very variable species and is grown in Europe for hay and found in meadows, pastures, moors and open woodlands.

Sweet vernal grass is native and common throughout most of Europe, western North Africa, Asia Minor, northern Asia and Japan. It has also been introduced in North America where it grows in many northern states.

Sweet vernal grass flowers in spring and summer.

A moderate cross-reactivity seems to exist to other important species such as Timothy (g6), Cocksfoot (g3), Rye-grass (g5) and Meadow grass (g8) (72).

Phadebas RAST®/Phadezym RAST® allergen g1 is acknowledged to be highly sensitive and specific (51).

References: 51, 72

Further reading: 2, 3, 4, 5, 6, 7, 8, 9, 10, 11, 12, 13, 14, 15, 16, 17, 18, 19, 20

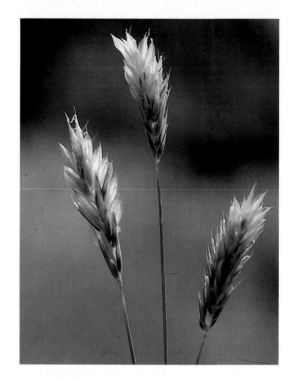

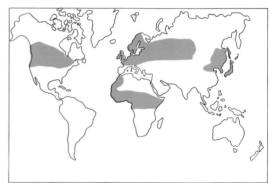

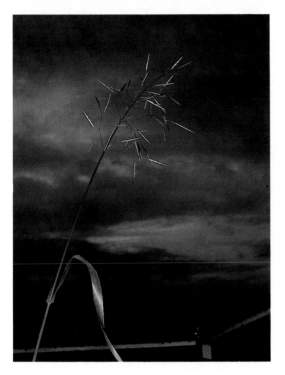

Brome grass is a sod-forming plant which resists trampling making it excellent for grazing and soil conservation. Once it is established, it has no equal as a pasture or hay grass and is both nutritious and palatable.

Brome grass is native to Europe, China and Siberia and was introduced in North America in the 1880's where it has since been cultivated in the northern regions of the US.

Brome grass flowers beginning in July and finishing in September.

Like Johnson grass, (g10) the individual allergenic compounds in Brome grass differ greatly from those of Timothy (g6) (145), indicating low or non-existing cross-reactivity to commonly found grass species.

References: 145

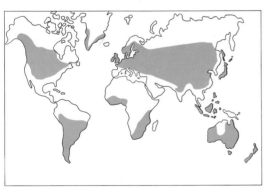

Rye is widely cultivated for its grain and as a valuable spring forage. The grain is ground into a flour for making black bread, crisp bread, whisky, gin and beer and the dried grass is used for roof-thatching as well as animal fodder.

Rye is cultivated in Central and East Europe and Russia and North America. It can be grown further north than any other cereal crop though its importance is on the decline. Today's rye is probably derived from *S.montanum Guss* which is native in the mountains of southwestern Asia.

Rye flowers in early summer giving rise to the well-known "smoke" when the rye pollen is released in great masses. Cross-reactivity to Brome grass (g11) and Cultivated wheat (g15) is suggested (72). *Secale* and *Triticum* are often crossed for agricultural purposes. An ALLERGO-DISCS® is also available for Wild rye, *Elymus triticoides,* g70.

Phadebas RAST®/Phadezym RAST® allergen g12 is acknowledged to be highly sensitive and specific (146).

References: 72, 146

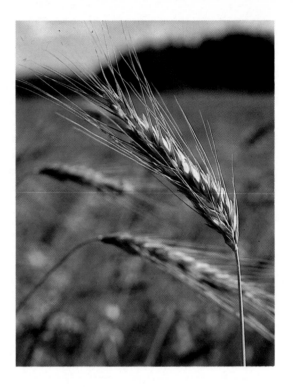

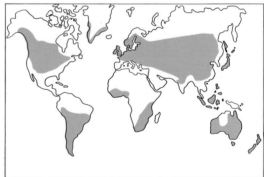

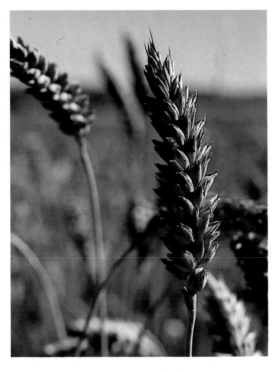

Cultivated wheat provides the staple food for about one third of the world's population. Wheat played such a large role in the days of the Romans that the empire was known as the ''Wheat empire''. The availability of wheat for food was considered a sign of a highly civilized society.

This widely cultivated and very important cereal is grown in temperate and subtropical regions all over the world. Wheat covers about 50 % of the total area sown with grain crops in Europe. The major wheat-growing areas are Canada, the USA, southern USSR, north and central China, India, Argentina and southwest Australia.

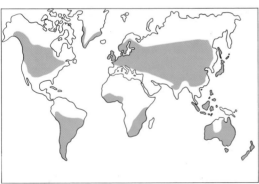

Cultivated winter wheat flowers in midsummer, and spring wheat flowers in late summer.

Many varieties of wheat are cultivated, such as durum and Polish wheat. All are closely related, thus having a high cross-reactivity to each other (72). *Triticum* and species of *Secale* have a tendency to hybridize making it difficult to identify the genera. There is only a slight degree of cross-reactivity to common grasses such as Timothy (g6) and Rye-grass (g5) (72).

References: 72

This is a creeping low-growing, greyish grass, one of about seven species of the genus *Cynodon*. It is the most common tropical lawn grass especially in dry areas and an important pasture grass in the southern US. It is a sod-forming turf grass and spreads rapidly when cultivated. It is considered to be one of the most allergenic grasses. In an American allergy survey, Bermuda grass was shown to cause the highest incidence of sensitivity among grass allergens (21).

Bermuda grass is found in much of Europe though not Scandinavia, in Ireland, Poland, South Africa, Australia, India, USA and Japan. It probably originated in India. It is the dominant forage grass of Brazil.

Bermuda grass flowers in North America from April/May to September/October. Around the Mediterranean, blooming occurs from May to August.

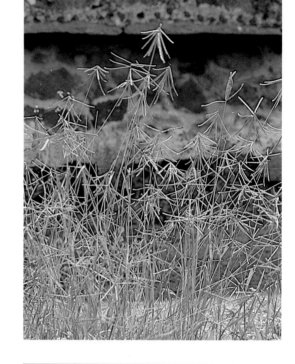

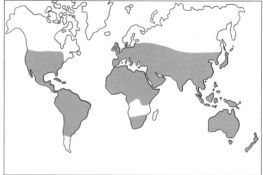

Bermuda grass shows a moderate cross-reactivity to Johnson grass (g10) and Bahia grass (g17) but only a very limited relation to other common but more distantly related grasses such as Rye-grass (g5) and Timothy (g6) (72).

Phadebas RAST®/Phadezym RAST® allergen g2 is acknowledged to be highly sensitive and specific (21).

References: 21, 72

Further reading: 3, 5, 6, 7, 10, 13, 14, 16, 22, 27, 28, 29, 31, 33, 36, 37, 39, 40, 41, 42, 43, 44, 45, 46, 47, 48, 49, 91

Bahia grass is grown for pastures and soil conservation. It reproduces by seeds and runners. It is a warm season grass and forms dense tufts acting as a pasture grass in the US and fodder in Mexico. *Paspalum* has about 400 species. The name *Paspalum* comes from the Greek word Paspalos, a kind of cereal.

Bahia grass is commonly distributed in the warmer parts of the western hemisphere and related species are found in the eastern hemisphere. It is native to the West Indies and South America and introduced into the US. One species is especially important in India for growing on barren hills because it is drought-resistant.

Bahia grass flowers throughout the year.

Cross-reactivity between Bahia grass and Johnson grass (g10) can be expected (72, 364).

References: 72, 364

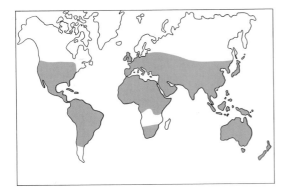

Johnson grass is a robust perennial growing in sandy and rugged soils. It is found along waysides and cultivated lands. It is cultivated for livestock feeding around the Mediterranean but can become a difficult weed.

Johnson grass is native to the Mediterranean area and is found in several areas of the warmer regions of Asia, Africa and the southern United States.

In the Mediterranean area, Johnson grass flowers between June and August. In other parts of Europe the season is from July to September. In the US, it usually flowers from May to July or in the extreme south – December to January.

Johnson grass is closely related to maize and cross-reactivity could be expected. The constituents of individual allergens in Johnson grass seem to differ from those found in Timothy (g6) for example, thus indicating very limited cross-reaction to species within the tribe *Festuceae* (145).

References: 145

Further reading: 143

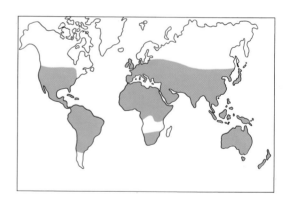

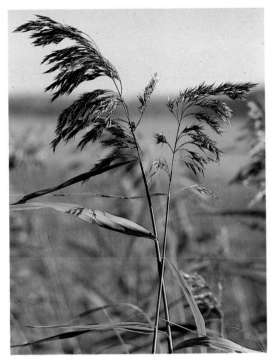

Common reed is a tall, robust, bamboo-like perennial grass often forming dense growths thus providing protection for nesting water fowl as well as preventing erosion. It occurs in shallow water along the shores of lakes and rivers, swamps, fens and road side ditches. The dried stems have been used for thatching, shelter, mats and more recently harvested for cellulose.

Members of the genus *Phragmites* grow in almost all of Europe, though not Iceland, and in warm and temperate climates throughout most the world.

The flowers develop later than in most other grasses and blooming often coincides with those of common weeds such as *Artemisia* or other members of *Compositae* in the late summer to fall.

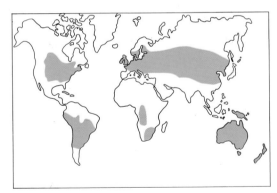

The allergens of reed pollen differ from those of the other common grasses. When screening a group of grass-sensitive patients with the allergen discs Common reed (g7) and Rye-grass (g5) a low degree of relation (r=0.50) was indicated (133).

Phadebas RAST®/Phadezym RAST® allergen g7 is acknowledged to be highly sensitive and specific (80).

References: 80, 133

Further reading: 10, 51, 121

Weeds

Despite the great number of weeds, relatively few are wind-pollinated or produce pollens of significant allergenicity. However, pollens of some of these weeds are among the most common causes of hay fever. There are about 50 000 species of which about 8 000 have "weedy behaviour". Of these, only about 250 species are considered problematic in agriculture requiring control. As a result of changing agricultural practices such as deep-plowing and herbicides some former "pests" are being threatened. The changing urban and rural tastes have created a market for seed companies who, for the home gardener, package "weed seeds" such as *Chrysanthemum, Solidago, Centaurea* and *Kochia.*

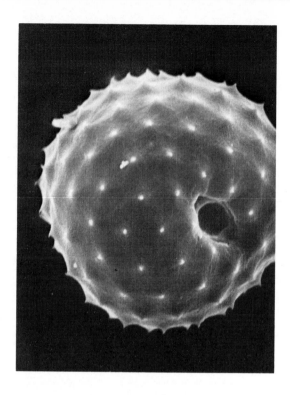

The geographical distribution shown for weeds is based on surveys of agricultural workers throughout the world. The maps indicate the areas where the weeds are of primary interest.

The allergen discs are grouped according to the family and sub-families as indicated in the diagram. Relationships between species can be better understood in this way. The schema is one of many examples of botanical classification but it has been followed throughout the grass, weeds and trees chapters.

All of the weed allergen discs are produced by coupling an allergen extract of a pure preparation of weed pollen to activated paper discs.

Organization of Weed Pollens according to genera

Weeds

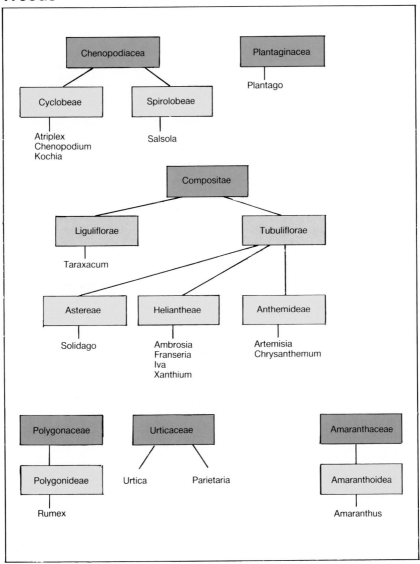

The genera followed by species are alphabetically listed in the text.

In the taxonomically complex genus *Amaranthus* some cultivated species are found. Common pigweed is grey-green with downy, oval-shaped pointed leaves. The flowers are a greenish-grey mixed with bristle-like bracts. North American Indians used *A.retroflexus* for flour and warm drinks.

Common pigweed is considered a serious weed in agriculture in Europe but also common in such diverse lands as Brazil, Korea, Spain, Mozambique, Mexico, Hungary, Germany, Afghanistan and America.

Common pigweed flowers in high summer and fall.

A high degree of cross-reactivity is suggested between the different species of the genus *Amaranthus* (72). Through correlation studies using a number of sensitive patient sera, cross-reactivity to Goosefoot (w10) was shown (362).

References: 72, 362

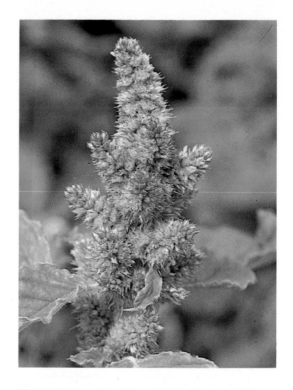

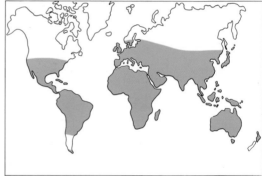

II:2

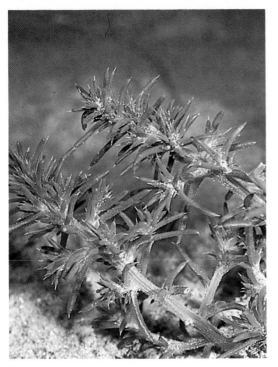

Saltwort is a prickly, usually prostrate annual weed of medium size. It occurs on sandy shores.

Saltwort is looked upon as a major cause of allergic rhinitis (190).

Saltwort is commonly found on the coasts of Europe, North Africa, Asia and North America.

It flowers in late summer and autumn.

Moderate cross-reactivity has been suggested between Saltwort and Firebush (w17) as well as with Scale (w15) (72).

Isolation and characterization of saltwort pollen allergens have resulted in the identification of at least two important allergens (191).

Phadebas RAST®/Phadezym RAST® allergen w11 is acknowledged to be highly sensitive and specific (80).

References: 72, 80, 190, 191

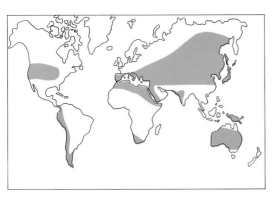

Atriplex is a genus of annual and perennial weeds and shrubs. A few species are grown as ornamentals because of their attractive greyish foliage. Scale often occurs along seashores and in saline soils especially in arid regions.

Scale can be found in the temperate and tropic regions of North America.

Scale flowers in late summer and fall and greatly contributes to the pollen loads of arid regions.

The different *Atriplex* species are closely related to each other. Cross-reactivity could also be found between Scale and Goosefoot (w10) as well as Firebush (w17) (72).

References: 72

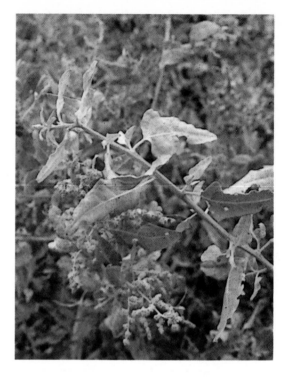

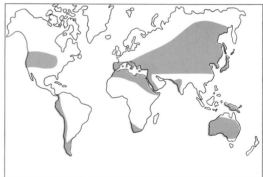

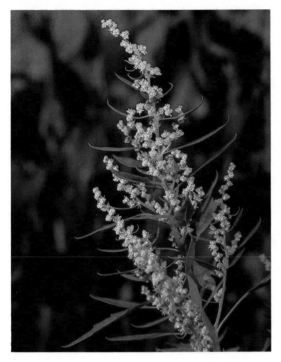

Goosefoot is an erect, annual herb varying much in size. It is very much a prehistoric and medieval food and medicinal plant. It is generally in open habitats, rubbish tips and on cultivated land. It is related to the spinach family and is vitamin rich. It can be cooked and eaten as a spinach substitute or dried, ground and added as a supplement to grain flour or given as an antidote against worms. *Chenopodium* comes from the Latin for goose foot which describes the shape of the leaves. Goosefoot was the first vegetation to appear at bomb sites in London after World War II.

Chenopodium species are tolerant of salty soils thus they play a role in the coastal flora around the Mediterranean, the Red and Caspian Seas, the central steppes of Asia, the edge of the Sahara, the pampas of Argentina, the South African Karoo, the Mulga of Australia and the alkaline plains of the southwest US.

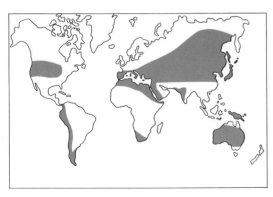

Goosefoot flowers throughout the summer and autumn. A full-grown plant can give-off as many as 20 000 pollen grains.

A moderate relation to Scale (w15) and Firebush (w17) should be considered (72).

Phadebas RAST®/Phadezym RAST® allergen w10 is acknowledged to be highly sensitive and specific (80).

References: 72, 80

Firebush is often cultivated as a bedding plant having small green leaves. It can grow into a small bush and towards the autumn its leaves turn bright red. It is a highly aggressive weed.

Firebush is widely distributed from southern France eastwards to Japan as well as in North America where it is a major source of pollen in the Great Plains and Great Basin.

Firebush flowers in midsummer.

Cross-reactivity is shown between Firebush and Goosefoot (w10) (r=0.60) (72, 348).

References: 72, 348

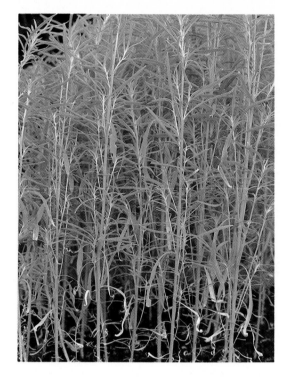

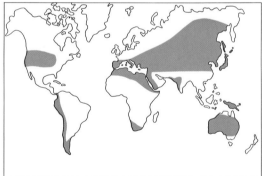

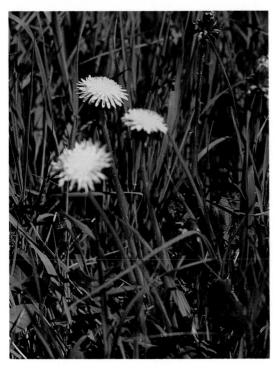

Dandelion is a perennial herb with deeply toothed leaves confined to a basal rosette. It occurs in meadows, lawns and waste places. Small children pick the plants when the flowers have gone to seed, make a wish and then blow, scattering the seeds in a thousand directions much to the consternation of weary gardeners. The small tender leaves can be eaten as salad, the roots can be ground as a substitute for coffee and wine can be fermented from extracts of the flowers.

Dandelion is native, common and often very abundant in most of the northern hemisphere. In countries such as Australia, Poland, Italy and Turkey it is considered a serious weed interfering with agriculture.

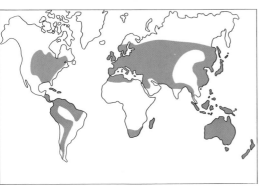

Dandelion flowers in spring and early summer, sometimes with a secondary flowering in autumn.

Many patients found to be sensitive to dandelion are likely to have been sensitized by other members of the *Compositae* family, like the wind-pollinated mugworts (w6) or ragweeds (w1, w2, w3) due to a close botanical relationship (72). The results from a group of patients RAST-tested with Dandelion and Mugwort (w6) confirm such a moderate cross-reactivity (r=0.9) (87).

Phadebas RAST®/Phadezym RAST® allergen w8 is acknowledged to be highly sensitive and specific (161).

References: 72, 87, 161

Further reading: 7, 98, 121, 174

Golden rod is a perennial weed
with yellow flowers which occurs in
dry woods and grasslands, on
rocks, hedgebanks and dunes.
Some species within the genus are
cultivated as ornamentals and are
very hardy. American Indians
ground the leaves and applied the
salve to rattlesnake bites.

Solidago encompasses about 90
species most of which are in North
America, though some species are
common to Europe and northern
Asia.

Golden rod flowers from mid- to
late summer.

Cross-reactivity is suggested
between different species of t he
genus *Solidago* as well as to *Aster*
and *Bellis* (72, 94).

References: 72, 94

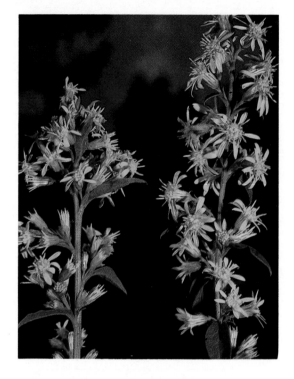

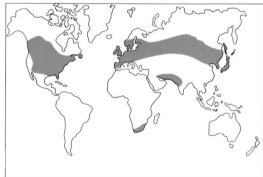

Common ragweed is a tall, branched annual weed. It occurs in dry fields and pastures, roadsides and waste places.

Common ragweed together with Giant ragweed (w3) is looked upon as the most troublesome species of the ragweeds in North America, inducing pollinosis and asthmatic symptoms. It is also a serious source of pollinosis in Japan.

Common ragweed is native to North America, but can also be found in Canada, Japan and Australia. Seeds have found their way into Old World sites probably as a result of the export of contaminated grain. It is a prime cause of allergy in the US though a ragweed pollen season is recognized in the upper Rhône valley, the Balkan states and the Krasnodar district of the USSR.

Common ragweed flowers in late summer and autumn. At its peak it can release up to 1 000 pollen grains per cubic metre in early September.

Common ragweed is closely related to both False ragweed (w4), Rough marshelder (w16) and Cocklebur (w13) and a large extent of cross-reactivity can be expected (72).

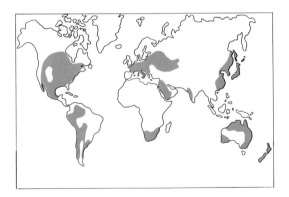

Phadebas RAST®/Phadezym RAST® allergen w1 is acknowledged to be highly sensitive and specific (149).

References: 72, 149

Further reading: 7, 33, 39, 55, 69, 74, 101, 155, 157, 159

Western ragweed is a perennial weed with a creeping rootstock. It occurs on plains and prairies, but also along roadsides and waste places. It spreads rapidly and becomes quite a pest especially when it invades cultivated lands and pastures. If dairy cows eat it, their milk becomes bitter.

Western ragweed is native to North America. Its range is extensive but is only significant in the Great Plains and Great Basin in the US. It is also common in Australia and Mauritania.

Western ragweed flowers from midsummer to autumn.

Moderate cross-reactivity to Common ragweed (w1) has been indicated (72).

References: 72

Further reading: 33, 39, 69, 155

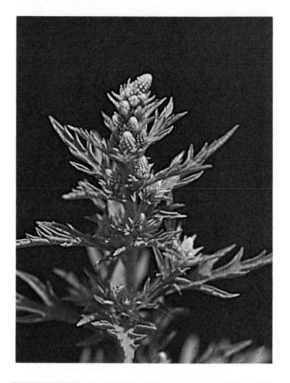

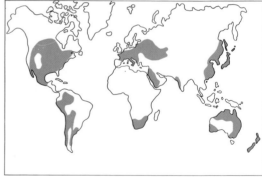

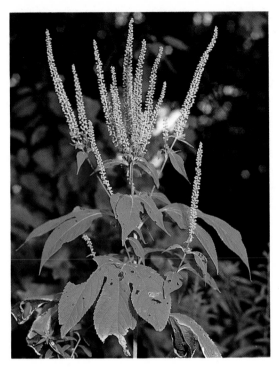

Giant ragweed is a tall, often 2 metres or more, coarse and unsightly plant. It can be found on low grounds and along side streams, often in waste places.

Giant ragweed is native to North America and is most abundant along the flood plains and southeastern rivers. In the Mississippi Delta it can form vast stands. It can also be found in Japan.

Giant ragweed flowers from late summer to autumn.

Cross-reactivity with Common and Western ragweed (w1 and w2) False ragweed (w4), Rough marshelder (w16) and Cocklebur (w13) can be expected. (72).

Phadebas RAST®/Phadezym RAST® allergen w3 is acknowledged to be highly sensitive and specific (7, 33, 39, 55, 69, 101).

References: 7, 33, 39, 55, 69, 72, 101, 155

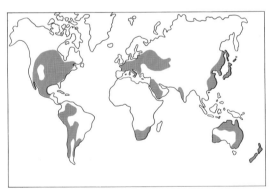

Compositae, Tubuliflorae, Heliantheae
w4 False ragweed *Franseria acanthicarpa*

False ragweed is a branching, annual weed, similar to the genus *Ambrosia.* Sandy soil, river bottoms and occasionally along roadsides are sites for false ragweed. This weed is considered to be a major source of pollen allergy in the US.

False ragweed grows almost over all the United States. Related species are found in Mexico, Hawaii and Australia.

False ragweed flowers from midsummer to autumn.

A certain degree of cross-reactivity is suggested between the true ragweeds and false ragweed (72). Low levels of antigen E, the major allergen in the true ragweed species, may contribute to this cross-reactivity (160, 82).

Phadebas RAST®/Phadezym RAST® allergen w4 is acknowledged to be highly sensitive and specific (80).

References: 72, 80, 82, 160

Further reading: 7, 33

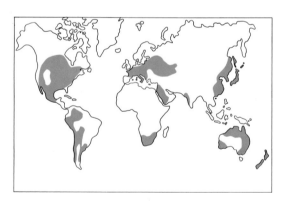

Rough marshelder is an annual weed which can grow up to 2 metres in height. It grows in wet, marshy areas, abused native ranges and low-vigour pastures. It has an odour like ragweed and can be mistaken for that weed.

Although some species of the genus *Iva* have been introduced in other parts of the world, most are found in the North American states of Texas, Louisiana, Missisippi, Oklahoma and Nebraska. It rivals ragweed pollen in the Missisippi Delta. Related species are found in Canada and Australia.

Rough marshelder flowers in the late summer and fall.

Correlation studies indicate a certain degree of relation (r=0.48) to Common ragweed (w1) (360). A moderate relation to False ragweed (w4) and Cocklebur (w13) can be expected (72).

References: 72, 360

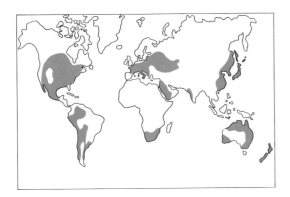

Cocklebur is an erect, often branching, annual, grey-green herb, up to 8 decimetres, with a slightly ridged stem. It occurs in waste places, fields, flood plains and beaches. It is poisonous during the two-leafed stage. The burrs often become tangled in the fur of grazing animals thus aiding distribution of the species to the detriment of the herder because the skins will not fetch the market price.

Cocklebur is a small New World genus, widespread in the American tropics and in Europe.

Cocklebur flowers from summer to late fall.

The genus *Xanthium* is related to the ragweeds (w1-w3) and Rough marshelder (w16) which are persistent hay fever species (72).

Phadebas RAST®/Phadezym RAST® allergen w13 is acknowledged to be highly sensitive and specific (80, 99).

References: 72, 80, 99

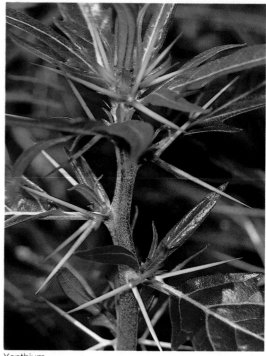

Xanthium

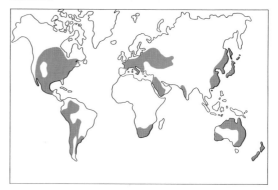

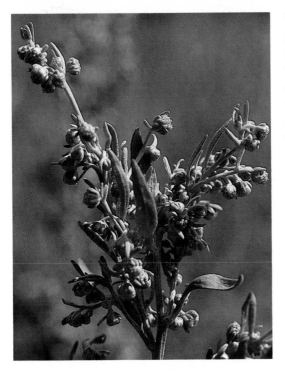

Wormwood is a medium-sized perennial plant with small yellow flowers. It is often seen as one of the only surviving plants in drought areas. This was used as a spice in medicinal concoctions in the olden days. In northern Europe, it was found in the flower beds in front of peasants' cottages ready to be picked. The weed has been used in the preparation of various liqueurs and aperitifs. It was a symbol of death among the Vikings and of victory for the Romans.

Wormwood is native and common in temperate Europe, the Soviet Union and found in America.

Wormwood flowers in late summer.

Cross-reactivity could be expected to a high degree to closely related species within the genus *Artemisia* but also to other genera of the tribe such as Marguerite (w7) (72).

Phadebas RAST®/Phadezym RAST® allergen w5 is acknowledged to be highly sensitive and specific (161).

References: 72, 161

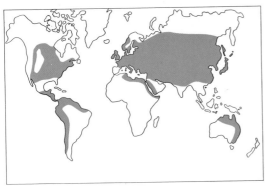

Mugwort is a coarse perennial weed which can be found in waste places, roadsides and shores. It is often seen in towns and villages. The word *Artemisia* comes from the Olympian goddess, who was associated with the Roman goddess Diana, also called the Goddess of nature. It is difficult to find a land in the northern hemisphere which is not blessed or beset by *Artemisia vulgaris.*

Mugwort is common in Europe, North America and Asia except for the northernmost parts.

Mugwort flowers during late summer and autumn.

Cross-reactivity could be expected to other species within the genus *Artemisia* as well as to Marguerite (w7) in the same tribe (72).

References: 72

Further reading: 4, 7, 102, 113, 161, 167, 168

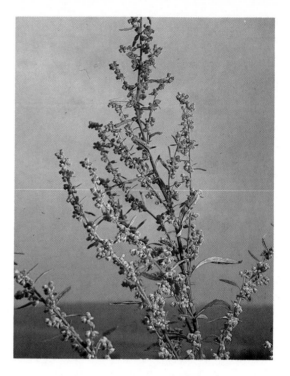

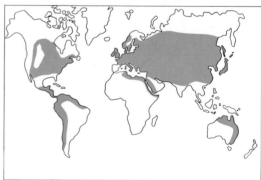

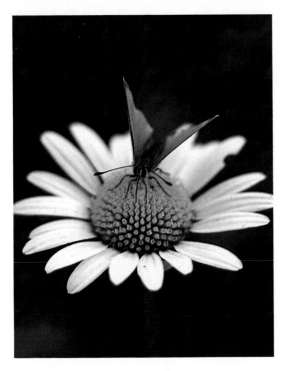

Marguerite is a perennial flower with usually simple flowering stems and few leaves. Traditionally the flower was used as a medicinal herb similar to camomile and is sometimes cultivated for ornamental reasons. In many lands, children have a game where they pull away the odd-numbered petals from the pistil to see if another person "loves me" or "loves me not".

Marguerite is found in Europe, Asia, North America, parts of South America, Australia and New Zealand.

Marguerite flowers in the high summer.

Cross-reactivity between the different species of the genus *Chrysanthemum* and Wormwood (w5) and Mugwort (w6) is suggested (72).

Phadebas RAST®/Phadezym RAST® allergen w7 is acknowledged to be highly sensitive and specific (161).

References: 72, 161

Further reading: 55, 94, 98, 121, 174

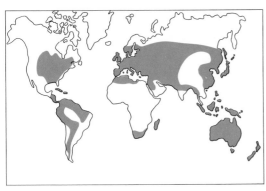

English plantain is a perennial weed of moderate size, which can be found in meadows or other grassy places, sometimes by roads. Members of the family have no known economic uses though in the olden days, potions made of plantain leaves were thought to aid in healing wounds and asthma. An ALLERGO-DISCS® for *Plantago ovata (psyllium)* k72, Ispaghula, is available for testing occupational allergens.

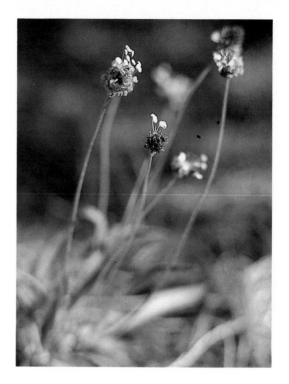

English plantain is common in most temperate regions, and is considered a troublesome pollen weed in such diverse areas as New Zealand, Mauritania, Italy, Canada and Ecuador, Belgium, Germany, France and the US.

English plantain flowers from early to late summer. It blooms particularly early in warmer areas.

The huge family *Plantaginaceae* (200 species) has a very high incidence of cross-reactivity among its members. Cross-reactivity to other plant families has not been shown. Using crossed-immuno-electrophoresis (CRIE)

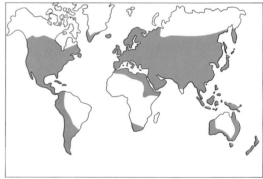

and RAST, 16 different antigens of which 6 may be allergenic were detected (184). Different surveys show a high incidence of allergic reactions, mainly hay fever, to plantain pollens (181, 182, 183, 184).

Phadebas RAST®/Phadezym RAST® allergen w9 is acknowledged to be highly sensitive and specific (39, 80).

References: 39, 72, 80, 180, 181, 182, 183, 184

Further reading: 4, 69, 85, 102, 239

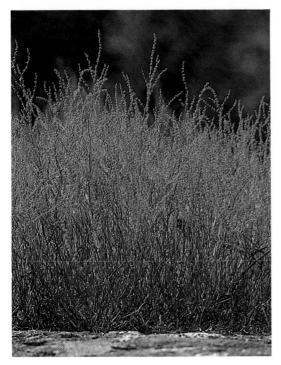

Sheep sorrel is a low-growing perennial weed. It grows on heaths, rocky soils, grasslands, roadsides, in poor, cultivated land and acidic soils. It is sometimes used as a pungent flavouring and can be bought at vegetable markets in France.

Sheep sorrel is a native and common weed in most of Europe, Africa, Greenland, Australia and North America.

Sheep sorrel flowers for most of the summer. The first blooming coincides with that of the early grasses. Sheep sorrell creates a reddish tinge in meadows in the early summer.

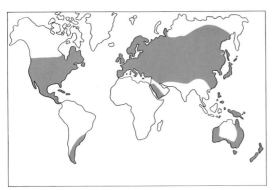

Cross-reactivity is found among different species of the *Rumex* genus (72). Sheep sorrel is often underestimated as a cause of allergic reactions especially in large cities (192). High and extremely high incidence of reactions to sheep sorrel pollens have been found (193, 194).

References: 72, 192, 193, 194

Parietaria is a more or less erect perennial weed, 30-100 cm. It has numerous oval leaves, 3-12 cm, and green flowers. It grows on walls, rocks and banks. It has been recognized as an important allergen causing symptoms of asthma and rhinitis in allergic patients. The leaves of *P.judaica,* w21, are about 5 cm shorter than those of *P.officinalis.*

Wall pellitory is a rather common weed in Spain, Greece, Italy and Israel and has been introduced in western Europe and Argentina. Two closely-related species are found in the US and one in Brazil. It is thought that the Romans first brought the plant across the Alps.

Wall pellitory flowers from early summer to late fall.

The genus *Parietaria* has about 10 species which are highly cross-reactive to each other. A close correlation exists between the species *P.judaica* and *P.officinalis* (89). In some geographical areas one species may dominate and IgE antibodies to only one of the species can be found in sensitized individuals. A high degree of cross-reactivity is also suggested to Nettle (w20) (72). Wall pellitory is an important allergen when looking for the cause of reaction in hay fever patients in certain areas especially in the Mediterranean area (195, 196).

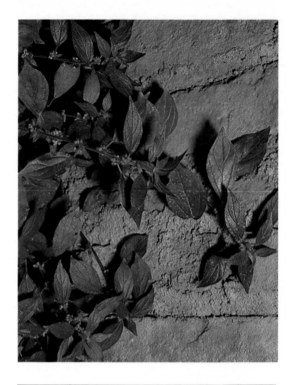

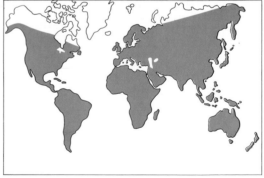

References: 72, 89, 195, 196

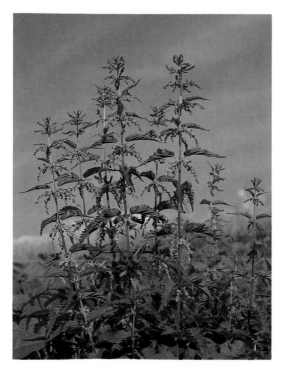

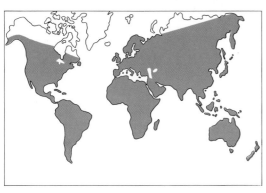

Nettle leaves are covered with stinging hairs which discharge their poison when touched. Contact with the leaves and stems usually causes a burning sensation and then rash. They grow to 1 metre and spread both by seed and by a creeping root system. The young shoots of these plants are used in soups, salads and tea. Nettle is found in open areas and near buildings especially in nitrate-rich soils. The fibre from the stems was formerly used in weaving textiles.

The species is distributed throughout Europe, western Asia and North Africa and has been introduced in western North America, Australia and parts of South America.

Most nettle species flower in midsummer and fall. Nettles have a curious pollination mechanism. When the sun shines on the curled young flowers, the filaments become taut and eventually shoot up so quickly that the pollen is released in a puff of smoke.

Cross-reactivity can be expected to Wall pellitory (w19, w21), which are taxonomically closely related weeds (72). Pollens of the genus *Urtica* are commonly found as a cause of allergy (198, 199).

References: 72, 198, 199

Trees

Many tree species produce large amounts of pollen which often induce symptoms of hay fever as well as asthma and conjunctivitis in sensitized persons. Trees account for most of the world's pollen plants under cultivation with the possible exception of timothy. Gymnosperms or cone-bearing trees evolved 350 millon years ago. During that period, the Devonian period of geological time, they were much more numerous and varied than today. Most of them are evergreen. Pine, firs, cypresses, cedars and junipers all shed enormous amounts of pollen. Patients can be sensitized to the pollen but also to the wood. The most troublesome trees are cypresses, junipers and cedars.

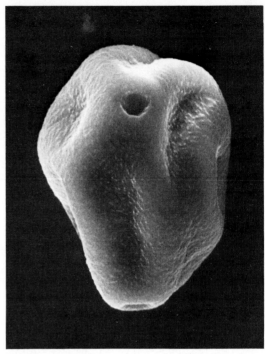

Common silver birch

Angiosperms are the flower-bearing trees and began their evolutionary struggle for only about 100 million years ago. In temperate climates most angiosperms shed their leaves, but in the tropics many retain the leaves and renew them periodically. Birch, alder, beech, elm and hazel shed considerable amounts of pollen in the late winter and early spring.

Trees have been central to human society first because of the discovery of fire, then shelter, utensils and as a means of transportation. The availability of trees has determined the migration of peoples and animals for example on the frozen tundra of Russia. The quests for firewood in the Sahara and Fertile crescent has hastened the encroachement of the desert.

Trees give each landscape its special character. The Mediterranean has the cypresses and olives. The eucalyptus is more closely tied to the Australian culture than any other land is to a tree. The pine forests of Canada impart a feeling of majesty and the vibrant fall colours of New England maples draw tourists from all over America. The "cedars" of Japan dot all of the islands and are extensively cultivated. The alder's silhouette gracefully reflected in a gently-flowing stream is typical pastoral scene in Europe. Scandinavia would not be recognizable without its birch forests.

In all cultures, trees have played a central role in folklore, being a symbol of female beauty and death, harboring both good and evil spirits, witches and fairies, mystical secrets and history of mankind. An old tree can summarise the climatic conditions for many hundreds of years when its rings and bark are examined. Birstlecone pine, *Pinus aristata,* in the Rocky Mountains at the higher altitudes has been used for calibration of C-14 dating clocks. This tree can live as long as 5 000 years. Trees are the oldest living plant in the world (as in Bristlecone pine) and the largest living plant as in *Sequoia-dendron giganteum* which grows up to 90 metres on the Sierra Nevada mountains.

Many trees have been transplanted to totally new environments and continents. Some have had better success than others. The geographical information presented here is only approximate for each of the genera. The classification system followed is one of many possible schemas. The trees are grouped according to the genus.

All of the Phadebas RAST®/Phadezym RAST® allergen discs for tree pollens are produced by coupling an extract of a pure pollen preparation to activated paper discs.

Trees

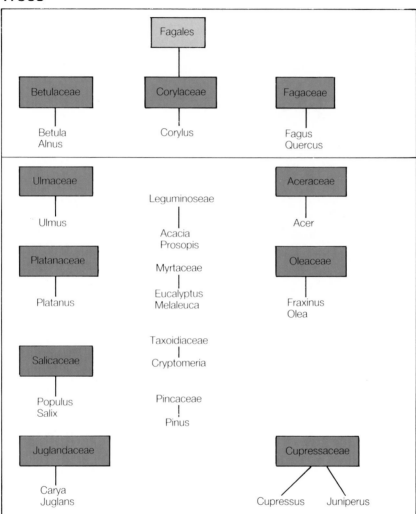

The genus and species are listed alphabetically in the text. Trees can be divided into two groups. The first represented by the order, Fagales, containing the families Betulaceae, Corylaceae and Fagaceae. These families are closely related and cross-reactivity can occur between members of different families within the order. The second tree group contains a variety of non-related families where cross-reactivity can be expected only between members of the same family.

III:2

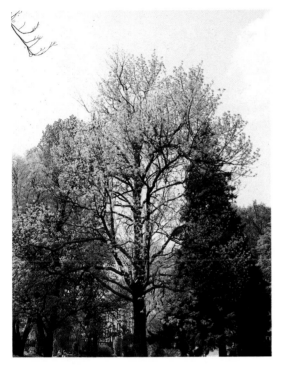

Box elder is a deciduous tree and can be up to 20 metres. It belongs to the maple and sycamore genus, *Acer.* The most distinctive character of the maples is the fruit which consists of two sections, commonly known as 'keys', each with a thin membraneous wing which remain on this species during the winter. The typical maple leaf is palmately 5-lobed and often as wide as it is long. The species *A.rubrum,* red maple, appears on the Canadian flag.

Box elder is native to eastern and midwestern North America where it is commonly planted as an ornamental and sometimes considered a 'weed'. The genus *Acer* consists of more than 100 species distributed throughout Europe, North America and Asia.

Box elder flowers in the early spring before the leaves appear.

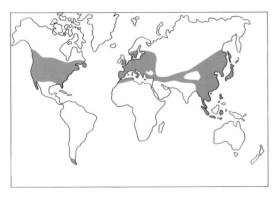

An extensive cross-reactivity among the different individual species of the genus could be expected (72). When comparing levels of specific IgE to *A.negundo* and *A.platanoides,* Norway maple, in elder allergen-sensitive individuals, 88 % of the patients showed a very high level of cross-sensitization (281). In a study conducted in our laboratories 53 of 128 patients with allergy to a variety of tree pollens had measurable levels of IgE antibodies to box elder pollen.

Phadebas RAST®/Phadezym RAST® allergen t1 is acknowledged to be highly sensitive and specific (80).

References: 72, 80, 281

Grey alder sheds its leaves annually and grows up to 20 metres. It is common in barren landscapes, woods and by lakes and streams, often in misty forests. It is used to enrich soil because of its ability to bind nitrogen. Alder has figured in mythology and folk tradition. Goethe wrote a summary of many beliefs surrounding alder in *Erlkönig,* the *Alder King.* Grey alder is found in both northern and central Europe though not Denmark, England or northeastern Europe. *A.glutinosa* grows in southern Sweden and Denmark. A closely related species, *Alnus glauca,* occurs in eastern North America, down to the Andes in Peru, Chile and Argentina.

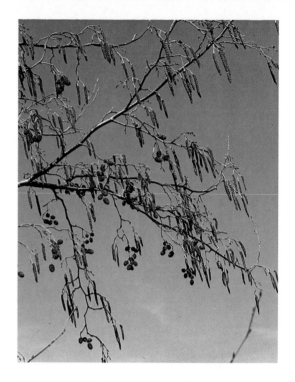

Grey alder has minuscule flowers and blooms in the early spring.

Grey alder belongs to the same family *(Betulaceae)* as Birch (t3). For taxonomical reasons, common, shared allergens could be expected and have also been found in these two species (200, 72). Cross-reactivity between grey alder and Oak (t7) has also been reported with Phadebas RAST® (208).

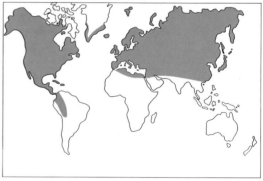

Phadebas RAST®/Phadezym RAST® allergen t2 is acknowledged to be highly sensitive and specific (201).

References: 72, 200, 201, 208

Further reading: 69, 167, 168, 203, 204

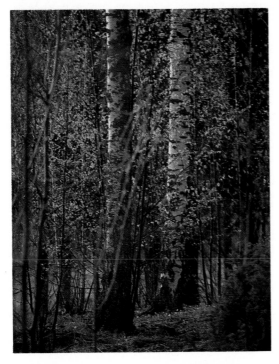

Birch bark and wood is water-proof which the North American Indians took advantage of when building canoes and wigwams. It has always had a special significance for festivals and rituals. It is never dark in a birch forest and in folk tradition birch is said to have a purifying effect. Silver birch is a single-stemmed, deciduous tree up to about 25 metres. The bark is smooth and silvery white, becoming black and fissured into rectangular bosses. Birch is a small to medium-sized tree found in woods, on heaths and often cultivated.

Silver birch is native and common in most of Europe, northwest Africa and western Siberia. It is the most common tree found in Scandinavia and the Alps and a potent pollen producer in those areas. Closely related species are found in East Asia and North America. It follows the mountain chain from North America down into the Andes.

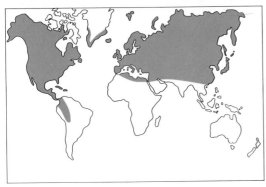

Silver birch flowers in mid-spring.

Studies of the different allergens in birch pollen indicate presence of major antigens which are also found in Oak (t7), and possibly in other tree pollens (200).

Phadebas RAST®/Phadezym RAST® allergen t3 is acknowledged to be highly sensitive and specific (80, 97, 102, 167)

References: 80, 97, 102, 167, 200

Further reading: 69, 101, 108, 201, 203, 206, 216, 217, 218, 220

Hazel is a deciduous shrub with several stems, 1-6 metres in height. It occurs in rich woods, scrub and hedges. It demands light and colonizes grasslands. Hazel is famous for its nuts which are harvested in the fall. It is also a popular wood used in inlay work and thought to have been cultivated in the Stone age. *Corylus* is the Greek word for helmut which describes the shape of the hazel – nut, also an allergen disc, f17.

Hazel is native and common in most of Europe except for the far northern regions. The principle commercial cultivation is found in Oregon (USA), Turkey, Spain and Italy.

The pollen develops in the late summer, overwinters, matures and is released in late winter or early spring. The first blooming appears after ten years. Hazel is the earliest blooming tree causing early onset of allergic symptoms.

A moderate cross-reactivity could be expected between hazel and species such as Beech, (t5), Oak (t7), Grey alder (t2) and Birch (t3) (72).

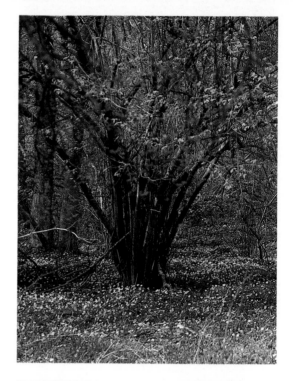

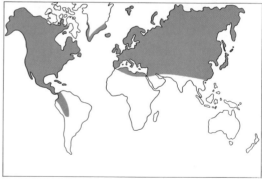

Phadebas RAST®/Phadezym RAST® allergen t4 is acknowledged to be highly sensitive and specific (80, 102, 201).

References: 72, 80, 102, 201

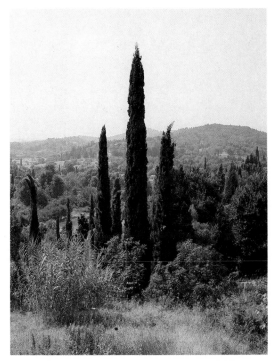

C.sempervirens is the cypress most often cited in classical literature. The tree has a perfect conical shape with a pointed crown. The scale-leaves and branches form tight, thick foliage. Cypress grows in dry areas where it has adapted well. The tree has been widely planted since classical times as an ornamental. It has often been cultivated in cemetaries, a tradition dating back to when the Greeks made wreaths of cypress to place on the heads of their sacrificial animals. The portico of St. Peter's in Rome is made of cypress because it withstands wear and tear. One famous cypress in Italy, north of Milan, caused Napolean some strategic problems. He planned his Italian campaign to avoid destroying the tree, now 5 metres wide.

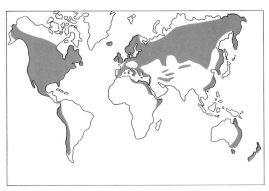

Italian cypress grows wild in the Mediterranean area and is distributed eastwards to Iran and Greece. It is planted as an ornamental in places such as Australia, New Zealand and Chile. It has been exported to China and India and along the Rhône valley in France it acts as a wind-barrier though it does not thrive north of Paris. But, it grows in Britain north to Edinburgh.

Italian cypress flowers from March to April. The seeds in the cones may remain on the tree for several seasons.

Cross-reactivity within the *Cupressaceae* family has been suggested to *Juniperus,* Mountain juniper t6 (72, 228).

References: 72, 228

Mountain juniper is a large, many stemmed shrub or a small tree, up to about 6 metres. In contrast to other members of *Cupressaceae* it grows at a snail's pace. It has persistent, aromatic leaves. It occurs in rocky soils in canyons, ravines, around rimrocks and breaks.

Juniper can live as long as 2 000 years and its reddish brown wood makes for long-lasting exteriors.

Mountain juniper is native in southwestern North America, particularly common in Texas. It colonizes grasslands and becomes a pest. The genus *Juniperus* is widely distributed in the northern hemisphere.

Mountain juniper flowers in winter (December and January). Male pollens and female flowers sit on different trees.

A high degree of cross-reactivity could be expected among the different species of the family *Cupressaceae* (72). In Europe, juniper *(J.communis)* seldomly causes sensitization in atopics.

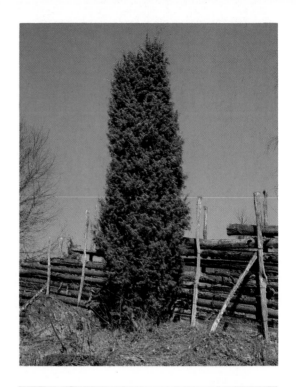

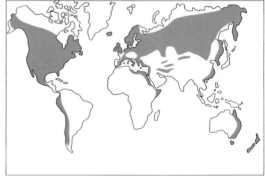

The flowering season of mountain juniper is closely related to the serious type of winter hay fever especially pronounced in the Texas, USA (228). It has been suggested that *J. sabinoides* causes allergic reactions in patients with no other sensitivities because of its chemical composition (342).

Phadebas RAST®/Phadezym RAST® allergen t6 is acknowledged to be highly sensitive and specific (44).

References: 44, 72, 228, 342

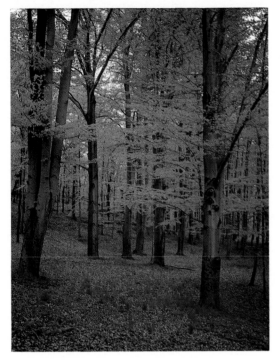

American beech is a tall deciduous tree up to about 30 metres. It occurs occasionally in woods and is sometimes cultivated though has not been successful in Europe. It is thought that the world's first printer, Johannes Gutenberg, used beech to make his plates. Of the broad-leafed trees, oak is said to be the king while beech is the queen. An ideal climate in Normandy has allowed the European beech to attain majestic proportions which possibly supplied the inspiration for France's cathedrals.

American beech is commonly found in northeastern America. In Europe this species is replaced with Common beech *(Fagus sylvatica)*.

The beech flowers in late spring.

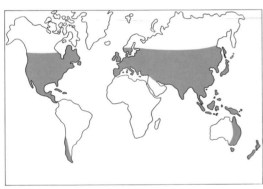

High cross-reactivity is often found among different species within the same family (72). Thus, of 54 individuals sensitized to Beech (t5) or Oak (t7) pollen allergens, only 13 patients showed specific IgE antibodies to just one of the species (208). This indicates a relatively high degree of cross-reactivity between species of the family *Fagaceae*. The extensive cross-reactivity within the genus *Fagus* has been demonstrated in our laboratories when measuring specific IgE antibodies in a group of beech pollen-sensitive patients. In 95 % of the patients a complete correlation between IgE antibodies against American beech and Common beech was obtained.

Phadebas RAST®/Phadezym RAST® allergen t5 is acknowledged to be highly sensitive and specific (80).

References: 72, 80, 208   Further reading: 206, 277

White oak is a tall, deciduous, noble tree with stout spreading branches. Oak has always been at the center of human society. Oak is mentioned in the Bible about 60 times and appears in all the literature from antiquity. More than 500 species belong to the *Quercus* genus. The availability of oak for shipbuilding has even determined the course of wars among sea-faring nations.

White oak is commonly found in north-eastern America and oak pollens are problematic throughout most of the US. Related species found are throughout the northern hemisphere. It flowers in late spring or early summer.

The cross-reactivity between members of the genus *Quercus* has been illustrated by comparing levels of IgE antibodies to white oak and English oak *(Quercus robur)*. When testing 64 patients with multiple tree-pollen sensitive patients the measured levels were identical (same class) in 78 %. In none of the remaining cases was the difference greater than one class (439). When measuring specific IgE antibodies to Beech (t5) and Oak (t7), members of the same tree family *Fagaceae,* 76 % of the patients had measurable levels of specific IgE to both allergens, indicating a high degree of cross-reaction between the two species (208).

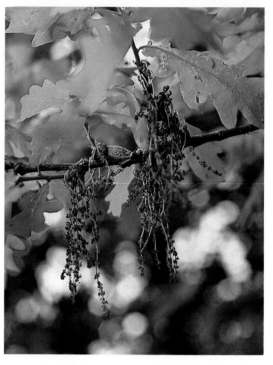

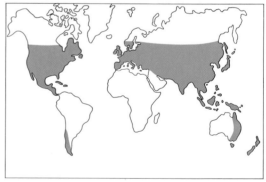

In contrast, to demonstrate the low degree of relationship between members of different tree families, specific IgE antibodies to Oak (t7) and Elm (t8) were measured in a group of allergic patients. In only 21 % of the patients could specific IgE antibodies to both allergens be detected (208).

Phadebas RAST®/Phadezym RAST® allergen t7 is acknowledged to be highly sensitive and specific (80).

References: 80, 208, 439   Further reading: 69, 168

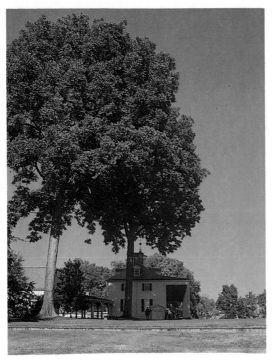

Pecan tree is deciduous, up to 50 metres tall, with a rather narrow crown. It occurs in forests as well as being cultivated for the fine timber and edible nuts. Oil from the nuts is an ingredient in processed foods, the manufacture of cosmetics and soap and is a drying agent in paints.

The range of pecan covers the warmer temperate zone and subtropical areas. It is very common in the southeastern US where it is native but also planted much beyond this range.

It flowers in early spring, shedding enormous quantities of pollen.

Cross-reactivity could be expected between species of the genus *Carya,* and on a moderate level to the genus *Juglans,* e.g. Walnut (t10) (72). The pecan nuts may also cause food allergy.

References: 72

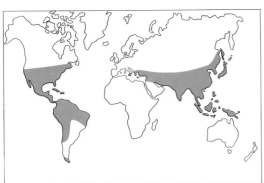

Walnut is a deciduous tree or sometimes a shrub, usually about 5 metres with a rounded crown. It occurs in woods and on mountain slopes. The largest walnut plantations are in California. *J.californica* is planted as a shade tree and is often used for rootstock for other walnuts. Its edible nuts are a delicacy and oils are used by painters and in soap-making. The hard wood is important in cabinet-making. The walnut pollens are often the cause of inhalant allergies and the nuts may cause food allergy (107).

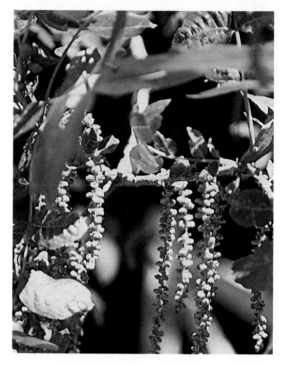

Walnut is native to California but about 15 related species occur in North and South America as well as in central and southern parts of Europe and Asia.

The walnut tree flowers in late spring to early summer first after 20 to 30 years.

There is a high cross-reactivity suggested between members of the genus *Juglans* (72).

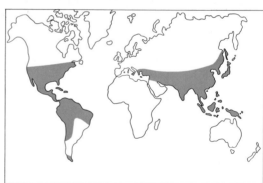

Phadebas RAST®/Phadezym RAST® allergen t10 is acknowledged to be highly sensitive and specific (80, 107).

References: 72, 80, 107

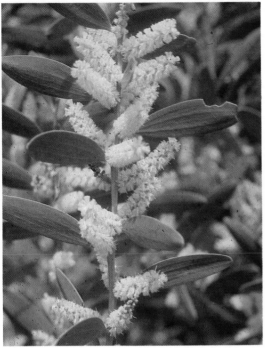

Acacia is called wattle in Australia following their use by earlier settlers for building huts of wattlework plastered with mud. *Acacia* is a large genus, covering more than 1 000 species many with thorns and spines. The trees are small, evergreen and fast-growing. They are planted for ornament but also for stabilizing dunes or eroded slopes. *Acacia* is a very characteristic feature of dry regions in India and the African savannah where they are called umbrella trees because of their shape. *Acacia* bark and wood are pregnant with oils and terpenes and are considered a source for occupational allergens (249). The acacia oil is used in the printing industry.

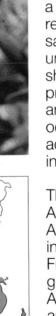

These trees are native to Australia, Africa and North and South America. They have been introduced in Portugal, Spain, France and Italy. *A.melanoxylon* is grown in large plantations in Australia, East and South Africa and Brazil where it is harvested for tanning.

Acacia flowers in early spring.

Extensive cross-reactivity can be expected among the different species of the genus and to some extent to species of the genus *Prosopis* (t20) (72).

References: 72, 249

Mesquite is a medium-sized deciduous tree or shrub armed with spines up to 5 cm long. The fruits are pods which are ground by the North American Indians and Mexicans for food. Its flowers are green and sweet-smelling but also cause hay fever. Mesquite pollens have been identified as an etiological factor in individuals suffering from asthma, rhinitis and conjunctivitis (250, 251). Large quantities of pollen have been recorded (252).

Mesquite species are found in arid regions of North and South America especially Argentina, South Africa and tropical Africa and Asia. It is one of the most characteristic shrubs of the southwestern US and Louisianna.

Mesquite flowers in early summer.

Cross-reactivity to other members of the *Leguminosae* family cannot be excluded (72).

References: 72, 250, 251, 252

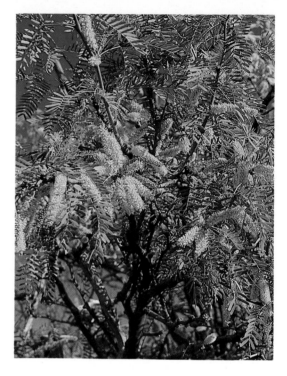

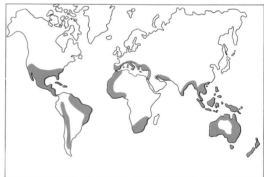

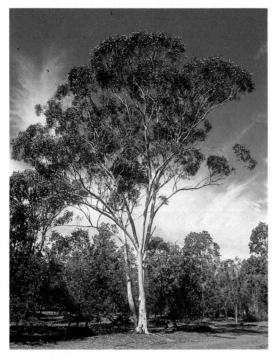

This genus consists of more than 600 species. The tree is evergreen and is one of the tallest trees in the world. Different species are grown for timber, paper production, oil yield as well as gum production. Eucalyptus is also an ingredient in tablets for soothing sore throats. It has been planted in swampy areas where its fast rate of growth demands much water thus performing a draining function. So, in some areas, it has indirectly aided the battle against malaria.

Most species are found in the tropics or sub-tropics coming originally from Australia. Whole forests have been planted in California and around the Mediterranean to help stem erosion.

Eucalyptus flowers in the tropics almost year-round.

A high degree of cross-reactivity among the different *Eucalyptus* species can be expected, and occasionally also to species of the genus *Melaleuca* (t21) (72).

References: 72

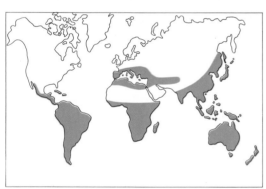

Cajeput-tree is a medium-sized evergreen tree or sometimes a shrub with a thick bark peeling-off in layers. Its beautiful flowers bloom in variable colours; whitish pink or purple. The spongy bark was used by the Aboriginies of Australia to make shields and canoes, for roofing and as timber. Melaleuca oil, used in medicine, is obtained from the leaves.

The Melaleuca is native to Australia and Malay. It is also planted elsewhere in the tropics and is rather common in greenhouses.

Melaleuca may flower during different periods of the year. In Australia it flowers from October to December. In California and Florida — from June to November.

Cross-reactivity can be expected among the different species of the genus *Melaleuca* and occasionally, to *Eucalyptus* (t18) and other genera of the family *Myrtaceae* (72).

References: 72

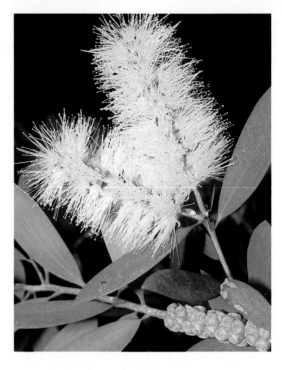

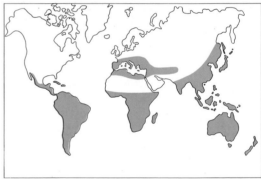

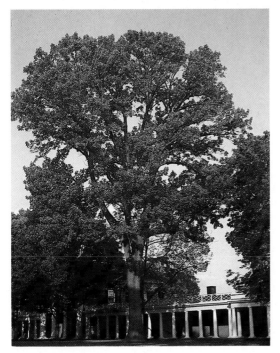

White ash is a tall, deciduous tree up to 40 metres and the most common ash. It occurs in mixed forests. The ashes are ornamental trees with handsome foliage. Their winged fruits hang in bunches throughout the winter and are shaped like keys which resemble helicopter blades when falling to the ground. They are important timber trees having light and elastic wood. The US exports ash timber all over the world.

White ash is native and rather common in eastern North America from Canada to Florida and west to the Mississippi. It is hardy and thrives in Europe. *Fraxinus* is a genus of about 65 species, which are distributed in the north temperate regions.

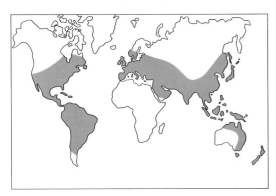

The ash tree flowers in the spring with clusters of yellow-orange flowers long before any leaves appear. It is one of the last trees to turn green and one of the first to drop in the fall.

A high degree of cross-reactivity can be expected among different species of the genus *Fraxinus* (72).

References: 72

Olive is a small, evergreen tree with a broad round crown and a thick and knotty trunk. It is one of the slowest-growing trees in the Mediterranean area. It is said that trees in the olive grove at Gethsemani were there in Jesus Christ's time. It is famous for its fruits and oil and by- products used in making soap. Its wood is used in cabinet-making as well as woodworking and jewelry.

Historically the olive tree has been cultivated around the Mediterranean and gives that region a special character. It was later introduced in North America, South Africa and Australia.

The olive tree flowers in the spring and the fruit ripens in the fall and winter.

Cross-reactivity between olive and Ash (t15) has been observed (72). At least 10 allergenic components have been identified from olive pollen (93).

Phadebas RAST®/Phadezym RAST® allergen t9 is acknowledged to be highly sensitive and specific (80).

References: 72, 80, 93

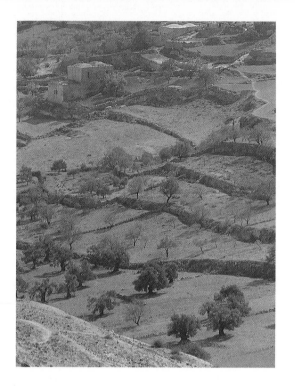

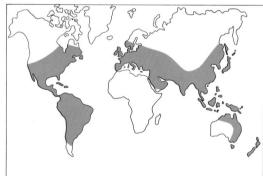

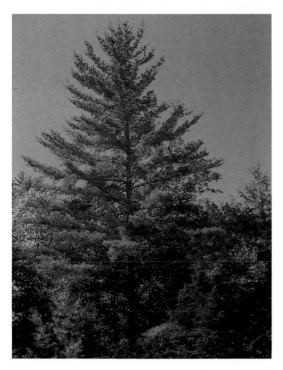

White pine is a tall coniferous tree with a blackish bark and irregular or flattened dense crown. It occurs in forests, is often planted for timber and survives dry, sandy soils or mountainous areas. It is becoming rare because this pine often becomes infected by a severe fungus disease. *Pinus* is the most variable, widespread and valuable member of the conifers.

Northeastern America is the native milieu for white pine. Cultivation was attempted in Europe but was given up because of the fungus disease. Of the 100 different species included in the genus almost all are found in the northern hemisphere, with 36 in North America. *P.radiata* or Monterey pine, has become the most important in the southern hemisphere. In New Zealand a 5-year old tree can be 7 metres tall.

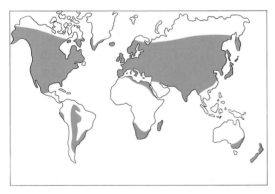

Most *Pinus* species flower in early summer. The male and female flowers are separate but on the same tree. The males form cylindrical catkins and the females form cones. The pollen count is often high (198).

Cross-reactivity is likely to be high among species of the genus *Pinus* (72). As could be expected no cross-reactivity has been found between this genus and other tree genera (white pine/birch, r=-0.04) (436).

References: 72, 198, 436

London plane is a tall deciduous tree. It is easily recognized by the bark which exfoliates in large flakes. It is very popular for planting as a shade and ornamental tree in cities as they do not suffer much from dust and smoke and can stand where other trees usually die.

The origin of this hybrid tree is uncertain. It is usually found planted in southern and central Europe to western Asia, North America, South Africa, Australia and New Zealand, especially in urban areas. In America the tree probably crossed with a native variety and thus looks different from the European species.

London plane flowers in the summer.

The different species within the plane tree genus are expected to be highly cross-reactive to each other (72). An allergenic glycoprotein compound has been isolated from the pollen extract of London plane (144).

References: 72, 144

Further reading: 198, 237, 239

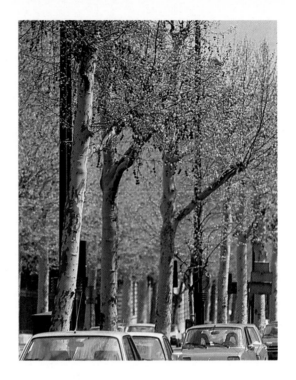

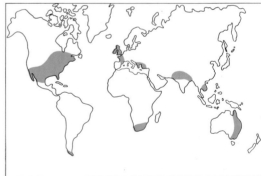

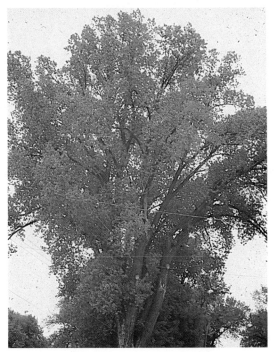

Cottonwood is a tree up to 45 metres with upright branches forming an open broad crown. It occurs in woods. Several species are planted for shelter and for use as a timber tree because of their fast growth. It is important for the paper industry and used for production of matches.

Cottonwood is native to eastern North America. It was brought to France about 200 years ago but was not successful. It eventually crossed with *P.nigra* to become a hybrid. The genus *Populus* contains about 30 species in North America, Europe, North Africa and temperate Asia. It does not occur in the southern hemisphere.

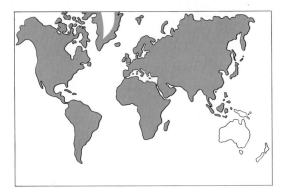

Cottonwood flowers in early spring. The pollen hangs on reddish catkins.

Extensive cross-reactivity could be expected between the species in the genus *Populus* as well as the species of the genus *Salix* such as Willow (t12) (72). The cross-reactivity studied between Cottonwood (t14) and Willow (t12) indicated a fairly high degree of relation (r=0.78) while Cottonwood (t14) and Birch (t3) showed no relation at all (r=0.13) (442).

References: 72, 442

Willow is a deciduous shrub or small tree, 3 to 10 metres. It occurs in woods, on shores, as scrub and in hedges. Some willow species grow very rapidly and are among the plants which are included for planting in extensive plantations as a source of energy. The wood is light and firm and yields salicine which has been used in head-ache tablets.

Willows are cool climate trees and are common in most of Europe, N. America and western temperate Asia. In eastern Asia it is replaced by related species. It is rare in the tropics and southern hemisphere.

Willow is one of the first flowering trees in early spring when it is important for bees as it is rich in nectar.

High cross-reactivity could be expected between different *Salix* species and to some extent to *Populus* species such as Cottonwood (t14) (72).

Phadebas RAST®/Phadezym RAST® allergen t12 is acknowledged to be highly sensitive and specific (80).

References: 72, 80

Further reading: 167

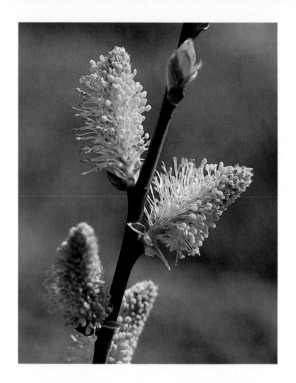

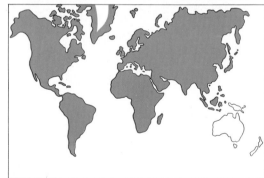

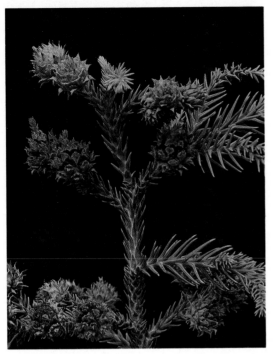

Japanese cedar, also called the Sugi tree, is an evergreen growing 30 to 50 metres tall. It grows in woods, often in pure stands, in rich deep soils in places sheltered from strong winds. Its needles shift from a pale opal in the summer to bright red towards the autumn. It is the most important timber tree in Japan where about one-third of the area under cultivation is devoted to it. There the tree is often planted in temple gardens and along roads leading to the temples. Japanese cedar pollen is the most common allergen for seasonal allergic rhinitis in Japan.

Japanese cedar is native to Japan and along the coastal provinces of China, and often cultivated in Europe and North America.

Japanese cedar flowers in March and April.

Cross-reactivity to other tree species is rare (72).

In a group (n=83) of hay fever patients in Tokyo, Japan, almost 90 % had measurable levels of specific IgE antibodies to Japanese cedar pollen allergens (244).

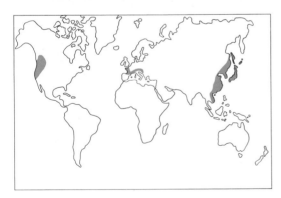

Phadebas RAST®/Phadezym RAST® allergen t17 is acknowledged to be highly sensitive and specific (244).

References: 72, 244

Further reading: 245, 246, 247, 248, 288

White elm is a tall deciduous tree up to 40 metres and is famous for its vase-shaped crown. It occurs in woods, hedges and by roads and streams. It is often cultivated and is a favourite avenue tree in cities and parks. The Dutch elm disease caused by a fungus originally found in the Netherlands, has decimated the elm stock in North America as well as in Europe.

White elm can be found mostly in forests in central and eastern North America where it represents a major source of pollen. The corresponding European species, Wych elm *(U. glabra)* and Smooth elm *(U. carpinifolia)* are distributed or cultivated throughout the north temperate regions. Fossils of elm have been found in Greenland and Alaska.

White elm flowers in the early spring while other species of the genus flower in the fall.

An extensive cross-reactivity is suggested among the different species of the genus *Ulmus* (72, 441).

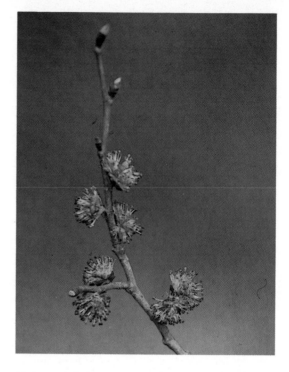

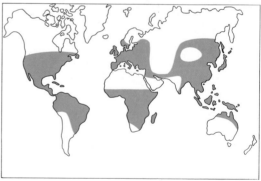

Phadebas RAST®/Phadezym RAST® allergen t8 is acknowledged to be highly sensitive and specific (69, 80, 168).

References: 69, 72, 80, 168, 441

Further reading: 107, 167, 198, 201, 232, 234, 237

Foods

That one man's meat is another man's poison is something that has been known since ancient times. Although most people can eat any food, in some cases allergic symptoms may occur when even a small amount of food is ingested.

Physiological and immunological processes serve to limit the amount of intact antigenic material which may penetrate the intestinal mucosa and gain access to immuno-competent cells or evoke immunological reactions. Enzymatic digestion degrades proteins in foods to non-antigenic fragments almost completely but some intact protein or antigenic derivatives can pass through the mucosa and stimulate immune responses at all ages. Other contaminants may cause reactions such as moulds on nuts or citrus fruits, insects on spices and antibiotics in milk as a few examples.

The term *food allergy* should be restricted to patients who have hypersensitivity reactions to a specific food with evidence of a specific immune response to the food.

The manifestations of food allergy are usually those traditionally associated with immediate hypersensitivity. Symptoms located in the gastrointestinal tract (vomiting, diarrhoea), respiratory tract (pneumonitis, asthma) and the skin (chronic urticaria, atopic dermatitis) systems predominate. Probably any food can cause an allergic reaction in susceptible individuals. The most common food allergens include cow's milk, egg, fish, shellfish, nuts, corn, cereal grains, citrus fruits, peanut and soy bean. An additional complication is that especially in processed foods many surprising ingredients are added such as coconut in packaged breakfast cereal or soy bean flour or milk powders in liver paté or even eggs in "genuine" mayonnaise. Or, patients may experience severe reactions upon entering a restaurant where shrimp or fish are being served. Medicines may contain flavourings which cause reactions. The wide range of allergens in the Phadebas RAST®/Phadezym RAST® panel permits effective identification of IgE antibodies to food.

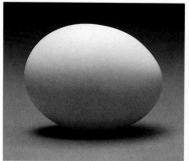 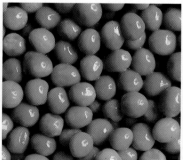 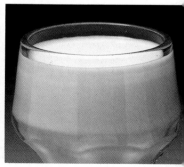

The figure summarizes the different types of mechanisms responsible for adverse reactions to foods.

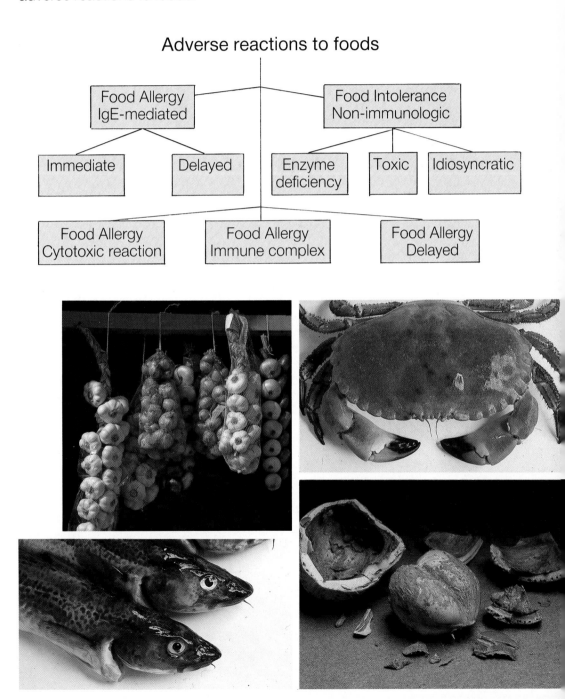

Adverse reactions to foods

Food Allergy
IgE-mediated

Food Intolerance
Non-immunologic

Immediate

Delayed

Enzyme
deficiency

Toxic

Idiosyncratic

Food Allergy
Cytotoxic reaction

Food Allergy
Immune complex

Food Allergy
Delayed

f1 Egg white

Egg white is one of the classical allergens responsible for early development of urticaria and eczema during infancy. Certain vaccines are grown on chick embryos and may cause severe allergic reactions in egg-sensitive patients when injected (264). An ALLERGO-DISCS® for egg yolk (f75) is also available.

Elevated levels of IgE antibodies to egg in 8-month-old babies have been shown to be predictive for allergy (272). In another study, patients with obvious egg allergies were judged on the basis of Phadebas RAST®, SPT and history. The authors concluded that RAST and SPT were useful supplements to clinical history (241).

Phadebas RAST®/Phadezym RAST® allergen f1 is acknowledged to be highly sensitive and specific (7, 201, 255, 256).

Phadebas RAST®/Phadezym RAST® allergen f is prepared by coupling fresh hen's egg white to activated paper discs.

References: 7, 201, 241, 255, 256, 264, 272

Further reading: 10, 105, 123, 239, 258, 261, 262, 265, 278, 279

f2 Milk

Milk is acknowledged as a major cause of adverse reactions in children. Babies fed with processed cow's milk are massively exposed to multiple allergens because the mucosa allows early passage of micromolecules (266, 267). Allergy to single proteins from cow's milk has been discussed and antibodies to alpha-lactalbumin, beta-lactoglobulin, casein (ALLERGO-DISCS® f76, f77, f78, respectively) and bovine serum albumin have been demonstrated (268). However, in many studies whole milk has been proven to be more effective than separate components in identifying milk-sensitive patients (269, 270). Patients allergic to whole milk were found to be only mildly allergic to pepsin digest of β-lactoglobulin in one study (284).

Phadebas RAST®/Phadezym RAST® allergen f2 is acknowledged to be highly sensitive and specific (80).

Phadebas RAST®/Phadezym RAST® allergen f2 is produced by coupling skimmed pasteurized cow's milk to activated paper discs.

References: 80, 266, 267, 268, 269, 270, 284

Further reading: 66, 69, 201, 239, 256, 258, 262, 265, 274, 275, 278, 279, 283

Allergy to fish is often combined with egg allergy but is less prevalent. Symptoms are often dramatic and even the smell of fish could release severe asthma attacks. Most patients react to all fish species and some may have an allergy to just one or a few. The cod allergen, ''allergen M'', is one of the most well-characterized. It is regarded as the major fish allergen, but it is not the only one present in cod and does not represent all other fish species. Testing for both Tuna (f40) and Salmon (f41) can improve the diagnostic capacity of the test.

Phadebas RAST®/Phadezym RAST® allergen f3 is acknowledged to be highly sensitive and specific (80, 255, 258, 285, 288).

Phadebas RAST®/Phadezym RAST® allergen f3 is produced by coupling pure preparation of allergen M from cod muscle to activated paper discs (255, 258, 285, 296, 297).

References: 80, 255, 258, 285, 296, 297

Further reading: 113, 239, 254, 291, 292, 293

Wheat, rye, barley and oat flours may induce allergic symptoms via inhalation, causing asthma, via food ingestion, causing gastrointestinal problems, or via contact with skin, causing eczema. Allergy to cereals is often developed in patients with extreme food allergy and is seldomly seen as a single allergy.

Hypersensitivity to wheat is found not only in infants but also in adults. Reactions are most often localized in the gastrointestinal tract.

Wheat, rye, barley and oat belong to the same group of grasses. A certain degree of cross-reactivity between these cereals could be expected (318). In a population of food allergic patients, 47 % were positive to barley, 48 % rye and 45 % to wheat which illustrates this relation (388). However, a specific sensitization to rye is not unknown.

Cross-reactions between cereal allergens and corresponding pollen allergens have been shown to occur (81). The cereals rye, oat and wheat are also available as pollen allergen discs, g12, g14 and g15. An ALLERGO-DISCS® (f79) is available for gluten.

Commercial allergen extracts of cereal grains have all been shown to contain substances which activate the complement thus possibly interfering with *in vivo* diagnosis (148).

Phadebas RAST®/Phadezym RAST® cereal allergens are acknowledged to be highly sensitive and specific: f4 (80, 258, 302, 303) f5, f6, f7 (80).

Phadebas RAST®/Phadezym RAST® cereal allergens f4, f5, f6 and f7 are produced by coupling extract of the entire grains to activated paper discs.

References: 80, 81, 148, 258, 302, 303, 318, 388

Further reading: 57, 143, 174, 239, 262, 265, 299, 304, 308, 309, 314, 316

Maize is the only cereal of American origin and it formed the staple diet of American Indians. The USA produces nearly 50 % of the world's maize. The crop is now grown widely in southeast Europe, Brazil, Argentina, Mexico, Africa and Indonesia. Maize is an important animal feed for poultry and pigs and is also a forage crop. It is used in starch manufacture and for whisky distilling.

Maize should be regarded as a possible allergen source from early infancy as it is an ingredient in infants' diets in many parts of the world. In a group of patients with food allergies, 38 % were found to have raised specific IgE antibodies to maize (388). A relatively low degree of relation is thought to exist between maize and the other cereals (f4, f5, f6, f7). However, a relation between corn grain allergens (f8) and wheat grain allergens (f4) has been seen (r=0,83) (434).

Phadebas RAST®/Phadezym RAST® allergen f8 is acknowledged to be highly sensitive and specific (434).

Phadebas RAST®/Phadezym RAST® allergen f8 is produced by coupling an allergen extract of maize *(Zea mays)* to activated paper discs.

References: 388, 434

Further reading: 147

Rice is the principal food for about 60 % of mankind. Rice hulls and straw are widely used as animal fodder and the straw alone finds many uses as a fabric. Rice has earlier been looked upon as hypoallergenic and used as a dietary food. However, sensitized patients have been diagnosed by measuring the concentration of IgE antibodies to rice (318). The incidence has been calculated in a group of food allergic patients where 34 % were found to be sensitive (388).

In one study IgE antibodies against allergens from both polished and unpolished rice were determined in patients judged to be rice-sensitive (259). No IgE antibodies could be found against polished rice. Thus, the allergens appear to be contained in the rice hull. Two protein fractions of rice grain have been isolated and shown to induce production of specific IgE antibodies (329).

Phadebas RAST®/Phadezym RAST® allergen f9 is acknowledged to be highly sensitive and specific (80).

Phadebas RAST®/Phadezym RAST® allergen f9 is produced by coupling an allergen extract of unpolished rice to activated paper discs.

References: 80, 259, 318, 329, 388

Sesame is grown extensively throughout the tropics and sub- tropics for its seeds. Sesame seeds have a pleasant nutty flavour and are used in making confectionery and as a garnish on loaves of bread. They are rich in oil, which is used as salad and cooking oil and in the manufacture of soap and margarine. The residue is used as cattle feed.

Sesame seed is more and more frequently reported to induce hypersensitivity. A surprising 38 % of a patient population having food intolerance showed elevated circulating specific IgE antibodies to sesame seed allergens (388). In several cases shock has been reported in connection with oedema and asthma upon ingestion of various sesame seed products (330, 331, 332). Another study reported severe anaphylactic shock after ingestion of sesame seed (333).

Phadebas RAST®/Phadezym RAST® allergen f10 is acknowledged to be highly sensitive and specific (80).

Phadebas RAST®/Phadezym RAST® allergen f10 is produced by coupling an allergen extract of the entire seed to activated paper discs.

References: 80, 330, 331, 332, 333, 388

f11 Buckwheat

Buckwheat is a large-leaved, annual herbaceous species. It is not a member of the grass family, and hence not a true cereal, but the seeds are used in the same way as cereals. The grain is used for human food in various forms from pancake flour to buckwheat noodles and baby foods, and it is also used as a feed for livestock and poultry.

Raised levels of IgE antibodies to buckwheat allergens have been recognized in atopic patients (371). In a food allergic population, 38 % showed raised specific IgE antibodies to buckwheat (388).

Buckwheat is also a potent occupational allergen. In a company which handles plant products, 13 out of 28 workers developed allergic work-related symptoms to buckwheat (77).

Phadebas RAST®/Phadezym RAST® allergen f11 is acknowledged to be highly sensitive and specific (80).

Phadebas RAST®/Phadezym RAST® allergen f11 is produced by coupling an allergen extract of flour from the entire buckwheat grain to activated paper discs.

References: 77, 80, 371, 388

Dried peas were once the staple food in western Europe, but nowadays, with proteins obtained mainly from dairy amd meat products, peas are harvested as an immature green vegetable.

The pea belongs to the same plant family, *Leguminoseae,* as Peanut (f13), Soy bean (f14) and White bean (f15), so cross-reactions between these cannot be excluded. The main allergic components have been isolated (378). The usefulness of the f12 disc for diagnosis of hypersensitivity in atopic patients has been well-established (174, 255, 291). In one study, 19 out of 24 food-allergic patients were found to have raised IgE antibodies to pea (34).

Phadebas RAST®/Phadezym RAST® allergen f12 is acknowledged to be highly sensitive and specific (80).

Phadebas RAST®/Phadezym RAST® allergen f12 is produced by coupling an allergen extract of ripe dry pea seed to activated paper discs.

References: 34, 80, 174, 255, 291, 378

Not only is the peanut a common source of protein in the diet in the US. It is also a common cause of serious anaphylactic reactions.

Peanut allergens often cause high IgE antibody levels in sensitized patients (258). The incidence of peanut- sensitivity in food-allergic patients was high (26 of 30) (34). It belongs to the same plant family, *Leguminoseae* as f12, f14 and f15, so cross-reactions may occur. A major peanut allergen has been isolated and partially characterized (445).

Phadebas RAST®/Phadezym RAST® allergen f13 is acknowledged to be highly sensitive and specific (80).

Phadebas RAST®/Phadezym RAST® allergen f13 is produced by coupling an allergen extract of raw, shelled peanuts to activated paper discs.

References: 34, 80, 180, 258

Soy bean is the world's most important grain legume and production is continuing to increase. The oil of the bean is put to many uses including its incorporation into salad oil, margarine and industrial components, linoleum and glue in the plywood industry where it is considered an occupational allergen (445). The protein in the bean is either processed into soy bean flour or incorporated into animal fodder.

Soy bean has long been regarded as a safe substitute for children showing adverse reactions to cow's milk. However, soy bean protein, like cow's milk is foreign for human beings. Therefore, no significant difference in atopic manifestations between children fed soy and those fed cow's milk can be seen (274). With its expanding use as a substitute and constituent in many different foods, a higher frequency of adverse reactions to soy bean can be expected. In a group of 24 food-allergic patients, 22 had raised specific IgE antibodies to soy bean (34).

Soy bean lectin has been suggested as an important allergen. Of 8 soy bean-positive patients, 3 were positive to soy bean lectin (317).

Phadebas RAST®/Phadezym RAST® allergen f14 is acknowledged to be highly sensitive and specific (269, 434)

Phadebas RAST®/Phadezym RAST® allergen f14 is produced by coupling an allergen extract of ripe dry soy bean seed to activated paper discs.

References: 34, 269, 274, 317, 434, 445

Further reading: 341, 342

Beans are cultivated in both the Old and New Worlds. The dried seeds of *Phaseolus vulgaris* are the haricot beans of commerce used in stews and in a sauce as canned baked beans.

In tropical countries the seeds are used largely as dry beans. White bean is botanically found in the family *Leguminosae* and cross-reactivity can be expected to Pea (f12), Peanut (f13) and Soy bean (f14). In many countries white beans are the staple food. Consumption of white beans is on the increase and must be considered as a food allergen of importance. In one study, 17 of 24 food-allergic patients were found to have elevated IgE antibodies to white bean (34).

Phadebas RAST®/Phadezym RAST® allergen f15 is acknowledged to be highly sensitive and specific (80).

Phadebas RAST®/Phadezym RAST® allergen f15 is produced by coupling an allergen extract of ripe dry seed of white bean to activated paper discs.

References: 34, 80

f17 Hazel-nut

Hazel-nut is popular in baking or eaten peeled and roasted. The reported incidence of allergy to hazel-nut appears high. In an allergic population more than 10 % of the individuals had pronounced symptoms after eating hazel-nuts (341). In one study of patients with unspecified food allergies, elevated specific IgE antibodies to hazel-nut were found in 68 % (34). In another study, nut-allergic patient sera were tested against 2 moulds, *Penicillium notatum* and *Aspergillus fumigatus.* One third of the patients were also allergic to the moulds indicating the possibility of a dual allergy (400).

It is a general observation that birch/alder/hazel pollen- sensitive patients react to the ingestion of hazel-nuts and to some extent also to Apple (f49) and other fruits of the family *Rosaceae* (341, 343). If this expression of hypersensitivity among such different members of the plant family can be regarded as true cross-reactivity is still in question. A pollen allergen disc for Hazel tree, t4, is also available.

Phadebas RAST®/Phadezym RAST® allergen f17 is acknowledged to be highly sensitive and specific (80).

Phadebas RAST®/Phadezym RAST® allergen f17 is produced by coupling an allergen extract from seed of hazel-nut to activated paper discs.

References: 34, 80, 341, 343, 400

Brazil-nut is the seed of *Bertholletia excelsa,* a large tree, native to South America. The tree grows wild in the rain forests of the Amazon basin. The trees are never cultivated but the collection and export of the nuts is a major industry. The nuts have a high food value, 60-70 % oil and 17 % protein. They have become a delicacy all over the world.

Although the incidence of allergic symptoms to Brazil-nut is lower compared to Hazel-nut (f17), it is still a frequently troublesome allergen (123).

The *in vitro* technique has been proved to be very effective for detecting the cause of immediate as well as late onset of reactions (123, 255, 344).

Phadebas RAST®/Phadezym RAST® allergen f18 is acknowledged to be highly sensitive and specific (80).

Phadebas RAST®/Phadezym RAST® allergen f18 is produced by coupling an allergen extract of seed of Brazil-nut to activated paper discs.

References: 80, 123, 255, 344

Further reading: 342

f20 Almond

Almonds may be classified by the presence or absence of a glycoside called amygdalin, into bitter and sweet varieties. Only sweet almonds are edible; they may be roasted and salted or made into almond paste or ground for use in confectionery. Both varieties contain about 50 % oil, used as flavouring and in cosmetics.

Almond is also a potent allergen. In a food-allergic population, 44 % were found to be almond-hypersensitive (34).

Almond has also been pointed out as a cause of *Acne vulgaris* (346).

Phadebas RAST®/Phadezym RAST® allergen f20 is acknowledged to be highly sensitive and specific (80).

Phadebas RAST®/Phadezym RAST® allergen f20 is produced by coupling an allergen extract of seed of almond to activated paper discs.

References: 34, 80, 346

Further reading: 123, 258, 288, 309

f23 Crab

In all, there are about 45 000 crab species which live in the seven oceans, in fresh water and on land. These 10-footed creatures are divided into about 30 families of the order *Crustaceae*. Crustaceans moult frequently during their growing stage discarding their out-grown shell for a new one.
Blue crabs are eaten just when they are moulting and have a soft shell.

Crab is a potent allergen, sometimes causing dramatic allergic manifestations. It may also be regarded as an occupational allergen in factory workers who inhale dust from seafoods (342).

To some extent cross-reactivity is likely to exist between crab and Shrimp (f24) allergens.

Phadebas RAST®/Phadezym RAST® allergen f23 is acknowledged to be highly sensitive and specific (80).

Phadebas RAST®/Phadezym RAST® allergen f23 is produced by coupling an allergen extract of boiled cleaned and frozen Atlantic crab to activated paper discs.

References: 80, 342

Further reading: 358

Shrimp is a member of the *Crustacea* order suborder *Nacantia* and has over 2 000 species. Shrimp is found in shallow and deep waters everywhere. The larger of the species, mostly in the Pacific are called prawns. They live on small plants and animals and have an odd habit of swimming backwards. Shrimping expanded rapidly after World War II because of improved processing methods. The United States is a major consumer importing shrimp from over 60 countries.

Shrimp is traditionally considered to be a highly allergenic food. Severe anaphylactic reactions are reported upon eating shrimps and also urticarial reactions after contact with shrimp. It may also be regarded as an occupational allergen in factory workers who inhale dust from seafoods. To some extent cross-reactivity is likely to exist between shrimp and Crab (f23) as well as lobster (ALLERGO-DISCS® f80) and crayfish. A major heat-stable shrimp allergen has been reported (380).

Phadebas RAST®/Phadezym RAST® allergen f24 is acknowledged to be highly sensitive and specific (80).

Phadebas RAST®/Phadezym RAST® allergen f24 is produced by coupling an allergen extract from boiled, frozen Atlantic shrimp to activated paper discs.

References: 80, 380

Further reading: 174, 258, 357, 358, 359

f25 Tomato

Tomato is second only to the potato as a vegetable in world food production and the most universally accepted vegetable in all cultural groups. They are eaten fresh or cooked. Relatively small quantities are marketed fresh, the great bulk being processed as canned whole fruits or juice, paste, ketchup or powder.

Tomato is probably the vegetable which most often gives symptoms in the form of urticaria or rash and itching in eczemateous patients. During infancy, adverse reactions following intake of fresh tomato are common. The incidence of allergy to tomato in different patient groups have been reported (262, 361). Tomato belongs to the same family as Potato (f35) but only a low degree of cross-reactivity has been reported (372).

Phadebas RAST®/Phadezym RAST® allergen f25 is produced by coupling an allergen extract of frozen tomato juice to activated paper discs.

References: 262, 361, 372

Further reading: 123, 258

f26 Pork

Probably China has the largest population of domestic swine but scientific breeding has taken place for the most part in Europe, notably Denmark, and the US. The domestic pig probably descended from the Eurasian wild pig *Sus scrofa*. A fat pig was worth its weight in gold long ago as an unrivaled energy source. Today, researchers are hard at work attempting to produce lean pigs.

In two patient groups the incidence of allergic reactions to pork allergens has been recorded between 7 % and 18 % (262, 361).

Aside from the usual allergic manifestations (asthma, rhinitis), fluid retention with diffuse oedema and weight-gain have been traced to pork allergy (361). Allergy to pork almost exclusively occurs in severe food-allergic patients. Game might be a good alternative for these patients, however, there is a great risk of developing allergy to these members of the bovine family as well.

Phadebas RAST®/Phadezym RAST® allergen f26 is produced by coupling an allergen extract of salt pork to activated paper discs.

References: 262, 361

The domesticated bovine cows seems to have originated from ancient India where they are much respected as life-giving creatures. The herders then moved on to North Africa and Europe. Cows were introduced in North America in the 16th century and reached Australia about 200 years later.

Allergy to beef is not very common and beef can luckily most often be tolerated by cow's milk-allergic patients. Beef hypersensitivity can occur as contact urticara in people handling beef or after ingestion as chronic diarrhoea, migraine, stomach ache, and other food allergy symptoms.

Phadebas RAST®/Phadezym RAST® allergen f27 is produced by coupling an allergen extract of raw beef to activated paper discs.

Further reading: 213, 365, 368, 374, 382

Carrot is an important and popular root vegetable, both for human consumption and for cattle feed. It is eaten raw or cooked and is often used to flavour soups and casseroles.

Allergy to carrot may cause urticaria and bronchial asthma but anaphylactic shock reactions do occur sporadically (366, 367). Vegetable allergens such as carrots are often heat labile and boiled carrots thus induce fewer symptoms than raw. The incidence of allergic reactions to carrot has been calculated to roughly 3 % in one patient group (123). Hypersensitivity to birch pollen has been linked together with allergy to carrot and Apple (f49) (369). The possible existence of a general plant (seed, fruit, leaf, root) allergen has been discussed (218, 371).

Phadebas RAST®/Phadezym RAST® allergen f31 is produced by coupling an allergen extract of frozen carrot juice to activated paper discs.

References: 123, 218, 366, 367, 369, 371

f33 Orange

Orange is by far the most important commercial citrus fruit. It was first cultivated in China 3 000 years ago. World production of oranges represents over 82 % of the world's total production of citrus fruit. Oranges are eaten fresh or pressed for their juice.

Orange is a commonly found cause of food intolerance occurring during childhood. In a group of children with food allergies, 5 out of 12 had specific IgE antibodies against orange (355).

In another study, the incidence of food sensitivity to orange has been calculated to be 4 % (123).

It should be kept in mind that orange contains many aromatic substances and colours which might cause hypersensitivity reaction by other mechanisms than IgE.

Phadebas RAST®/Phadezym RAST® allergen f33 is produced by coupling an allergen extract of frozen orange juice to activated paper discs.

References: 123, 355

Further reading: 258

Wild potato tubers were first cultivated by the Incas in South and Central America. The Peruvian department of the UN/FAO has preserved some 12 000 species of the primitive cultivated forms of potato. Potato was brought to Europe in the 16th century. Nutritionally the potato is outstanding as a food and comes fourth after wheat, rice and corn as a staple crop.

Eating potatoes seldomly releases hypersensitivity reactions, but peeling potatoes will often cause eczema on the hands and, in tree-pollen allergic patients, itching in the mouth, rhinitis and irritation in the eyes. Bronchial asthma, urticaria and Quincke-oedema are other symptoms associated with allergy to potato (374).

Cross-reactive antibodies have been proposed between potato and other vegetables as well as pollens (371). However, when comparing the immunological cross-reactivity between Potato (f35) and Tomato (f25) which are of the same family, a low degree of relation (r=0.22) has been reported (372).

Phadebas RAST®/Phadezym RAST® allergen f35 is produced by coupling an allergen extract of fresh potato, *(Solanum tuberosum)* including the peel, to activated paper discs.

References: 371, 372, 374

Coconuts provide the fat ration for about 70 % of the world's population. The oil is used to make margarine, soap and detergents. Desicated coconut consists of shredded and dried endosperm and is exported from Sri Lanka and the Philippines. Coconut milk, from the unripe fruits, provides a refreshing drink. Coconut is also used in baking, breakfast cereals and chocolate candies.

The allergy is common and all degrees of severity are seen, from itching in the mouth, urticaria to life-threatening anaphylactic shock. Allergy to coconut often appears in the early teenage years. In a clinical study, sera from 16 food-allergic patients were tested. Of those, 6 patients showed raised specific IgE antibodies to coconut (34).

Phadebas RAST®/Phadezym RAST® allergen f36 is acknowledged to be highly sensitive and specific (80).

Phadebas RAST®/Phadezym RAST® allergen f36 is produced by coupling an allergen extract of shredded coconut to activated paper discs.

References: 34, 80

f37 Blue mussel

Mussels are bivalue molluscs of the genus *Mytilis,* denoting marine and edible. Mussels prefer cooler seas where they attach themselves to solid objects or one another by threads. *M.edulis* has been cultivated in Europe since the 13th century and has figured in the diet in the cooler regions there.

Blue mussels, as well as other seafoods, are known to often cause hypersensitivity reactions such as urticaria and symptoms in the gastrointestinal tract. The time of year is important for the blue mussel's capability of inducing allergic symptoms.

A high cross-reactivity between blue mussels and oysters has been indicated in preliminary studies (363). Cross-reactivity between blue mussel and Crab (f23) allergens has also been suggested (r=0.71) (363).

Phadebas RAST®/Phadezym RAST® allergen f37 is produced by coupling an allergen extract of canned blue mussel to activated paper discs.

References: 363

f40 Tuna

Tuna is one of the oceanic fishes having great commercial value. It thrives in warmer seas where different species vary considerably in size and appearance. The classification differs from one authority to the next but it is generally agreed that tuna is related to the mackerels. Tuna has been hunted since ancient times but the overzealous fishing of our century has resulted in their being 'over-fished' both in the Atlantic and Pacific oceans.

About 50 % if not more of the global tuna harvest is canned or frozen for the US market. A medicinal contribution from tuna is insulin.

Although Phadebas RAST®/Phadezym RAST® allergen f3 (cod) is a highly suitable allergen for *in vitro* diagnosis of fish sensitivity in most cases, some patients may not show specific IgE antibodies to cod allergen M. Allergen f40 will improve the diagnostic capacity of the test.

In a group of fish sensitized patients, cross-reactivity between tuna fish and Cod (f3) was found (r=0.55) (354). Cross-reactivity was also shown (r=0.56) between tuna fish and Salmon (f41) (354). Scomboid poisoning due to tuna and related fish containing high levels of histamine resembles food allergy (318).

Phadebas RAST®/Phadezym RAST® allergen f40 is produced by coupling an allergen extract of canned tuna fish to activated paper discs.

References: 354, 318

Salmon are anadromous which means they migrate to the ocean waters as fingerlings to grow but return to the fresh water river beds to spawn. The Pacific salmon spawn and die whereas the Atlantic species makes several returns.

Allergy to fish is often combined with allergy to egg, but is not that common. Some patients may be more or less sensitive to different fish species. Thus, allergen f41 is a good complement to f3 Cod and f40 Tuna in fish allergy diagnosis.

Cross-reactivity between salmon and Tuna (f40) (r=0.56) and between salmon and Cod (f3) (r=0.72) has been reported (352). Interestingly, salmon has been reported as containing as much as 7.4 μg/ml of histamine (350). If true, this factor excludes the use of salmon allergen extracts for *in vivo* tests in order to avoid false positive reactions.

Phadebas RAST®/Phadezym RAST® allergen f41 is produced by coupling an allergen extract of frozen salmon to activated paper discs.

References: 350, 352

Strawberry, a well-known, edible soft fruit, is distributed throughout Eurasia and America, and is increasingly grown in warmer climates. It was first cultivated in France about 250 years ago using a hybrid of two American species. The fruit is eaten fresh or processed for preserves, canning and freezing.

Strawberry is a common cause of hypersensitivity reactions especially in young children. Many of these reactions may also be mediated by other mechanisms than IgE or induced by aromatic substances and colours found in strawberries. Skin manifestations are common symptoms in individuals sensitized to strawberries. The incidence of strawberry allergy was found to be at 4 % in one investigation (123).

Phadebas RAST®/Phadezym RAST® allergen f44 is produced by coupling an allergen extract of frozen strawberries to activated paper discs.

References: 123

f45 Yeast *Saccharomyces cerevisiae*

Yeast is an economically important fungus including several species used in brewing and baking industries. No allergenic difference has been observed between Baker's yeast and Brewer's yeast. A possible cross-reactivity between the food yeasts and *Candida albicans* (m5) has been reported (327, 379).

Hypersensitivity to yeast has been recognized more and more. Symptoms such as eczema, nasal congestion, asthma and rhinitis have been found (377). As many as 33 % of a group of migraine patients showed hypsersensitivity to yeast (368).

Phadebas RAST®/Phadezym RAST® allergen f45 is produced by coupling an allergen extract of dry yeast to activated paper discs.

References: 327, 368, 377, 379

f47 Garlic

Garlic is a small extremely pungent, onion-like plant which is widely used for flavouring in salads, meat and savoury dishes, particularly in the Mediterranean countries, the Middle and Far East and South America.

Garlic has been shown to evoke both bronchial as well as nasal and skin reactions (379, 380). For many years garlic has been regarded as an occupational allergen through inhalation of garlic dust (377, 378). Elevated specific IgE levels have been found in garlic-sensitized patients (377, 378). Laboratory testing indicates a certain degree of cross-reactivity between Onion (f48) and garlic both belonging to the *Liliaceae* family.

Phadebas RAST®/Phadezym RAST® allergen f47 is produced by coupling an allergen extract of garlic powder to activated paper discs.

References: 377, 378, 379, 380

Further reading: 223, 224, 242

The common onion probably originated in Central Asia, and there are references to its cultivation in the Middle East dating back at least 3000 years. Compared to other fresh vegetables onions are highly indigestable carbohydrates and intermediate in protein content. When onion tissue is wounded, an enzyme reaction releases sulphur-containing volatile compounds, which give onions their characteristic flavour and lackrymatory properties.

Historically, onion has been recognized as an occupational allergen usually responsible for contact dermatitis (381, 382, 383, 384). Onion may cause gastroenteric symptoms or other atopic manifestations may occur. A group of patients whose case histories indicated onion allergy was tested using different discs with red and yellow onion as well as garlic. There was a high degree of cross-reactivity among the three:

yellow onion — 57 % positive,
red onion, and garlic, both — 71 % positive (340).

Onions are rich in etheric oils and other irritants, which leads to questionable results when testing *in vivo.*

Phadebas RAST®/Phadezym RAST® allergen f48 is produced by coupling an allergen extract of vacuum-dried onion to activated paper discs.

References: 340, 381, 382, 383, 384

Apples can be classified into four main groups: dessert, culinary, cider and ornamental. The apples are used for cider, apple juice, wine, liqueurs, vinegar, as fillings for tarts, pies, and sauces or eaten fresh. The apple is also cultivated for ornamental reasons.

Apple allergy is frequently found especially in patients with immediate hypersensitivity to birch pollen. Approximately 50 % of the patients in a group with hypersensitivity to birch were also sensitive to apple, as judged by a history of symptoms, skin test and RAST (218, 286, 369).

Phadebas RAST®/Phadezym RAST® allergen f49 is produced by coupling an allergen extract of whole, ripe green apples to activated paper discs.

References: 218, 369

Epidermals and animal proteins

Dander and other animal emanations have long been known to be major sources of allergens. In recent years, the incidence of animal allergies receiving clinical attention has been increasing. This is attributable to the increased proliferation of fur-bearing animals in urban homes, rural areas and test laboratories.

Cats and dogs are commonly recognized as carriers of the most easily available allergens inducing perennial asthma and rhinitis as well as conjunctivitis in children and adults. Horse and cow allergens could be looked upon also as occupational, inducing allergic manifestations in horse breeders, stablehands, farmers and veterinarians. Occupation-related hypersensitivity reactions frequently occur among laboratory personnel exposed to animals such as mice, rats, rabbits and guinea pigs.

Exposure to animal allergens can occur in different ways. Hypersensitivity reactions may be due to direct contact or inhalation of dust particles carrying allergens derived from animal epithelia, saliva, sera or urine.

Common as well as species-specific animal allergens have been suggested because of cross-reactivity patterns seen in sensitized patients.

Investigators of animal dander hypersensitivity meet several difficulties. Skin tests are often unreliable and less than half of the positive skin tests may have clinical relevance. Traditional allergen extracts were prepared from a variety of unspecified sources such as whole pelts, epithelia (skin scrapings), dander or hair. Extracts of these different types varied widely in their composition and concentration.

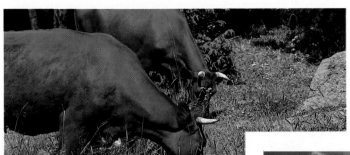

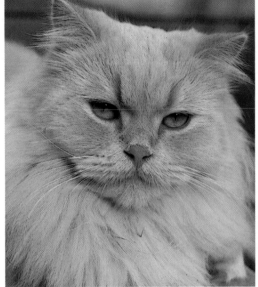

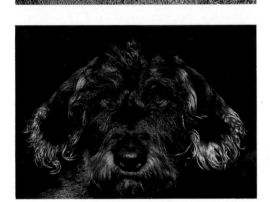

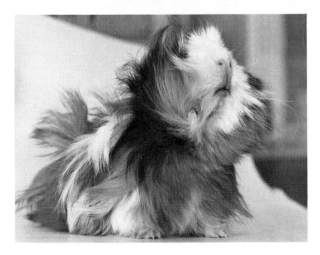

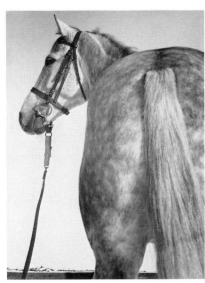

Cats are considered to be the most highly allergenic of the different animal species for most people (392), causing asthma and rhinitis. Allergens from different cat breeds appear to be closely related (393, 394). The allergens involved in cat allergy have been studied in pelt extract, saliva, serum and urine. One major allergen has been found, called cat allergen 1, whereas albumin and several unidentified proteins play a minor role (411). Cross-reactivity to a dog allergen has been shown (401).

Phadebas RAST®/Phadezym RAST® allergen e1 is acknowledged to be highly sensitive and specific (121, 201, 385, 386, 387, 390, 391).

Phadebas RAST®/Phadezym RAST® allergen e1 is produced by coupling an allergen extract of cat epithelium to activated paper discs.

References: 121, 201, 385, 386, 387, 390, 391, 392, 393, 394, 401, 411

Further reading: 23, 55, 101, 105, 395, 396, 397, 398, 402, 404, 405, 406, 407, 408, 409, 410, 412, 413, 414, 415, 416, 417

Immediate hypersensitivity to dog is well-known. Responsible allergens for the allergic symptoms could be specific epithelial proteins (408, 419, 420) or serum proteins (401, 419, 420, 422) including a protein, which biochemically and immunologically is closely related to a major cat allergen (401). A number of major allergens from different allergenic sources have been identified through RAST-based allergen assay methods as well as with crossed-immunoelectrophoresis (CIE) and crossed-radioimmunoelectrophoresis (CRIE) (101, 397, 409, 415, 424, 427, 428).

Breed-specific allergens have been discussed (431 , 432). In a comparative study epithelia from three species, poodle, boxer (German bulldog) and Alsatian, were coupled to discs and patient sera were tested. Of 115 patients, 67 % were positive to e2; 52 %, 40 % and 29 % for poodle, boxer and Alsatian, respectively (307). Only 3 patients of 115 were shown to have specific allergy to boxer epithelia not identified by e2. Thus, the e2 allergen disc is effective for testing a crude range of dog epithelia allergies.

Phadebas RAST®/Phadezym RAST® allergen e2 is acknowledged to be highly sensitive and specific (23, 97, 105, 385, 386, 387, 390, 391, 395, 443).

Phadebas RAST®/Phadezym RAST® allergen e2 is produced by coupling an allergen extract of dachshund epithelium to activated paper discs.

References: 23, 97, 101, 105, 307, 385, 386, 387, 390, 391, 395, 397, 401, 408, 409, 415, 419, 420, 422, 424, 427, 428, 431, 432, 443

Further reading: 121, 174, 335, 407, 412, 430, 433, 435, 437, 438, 444

Horse is known as a source of a very potent allergen. Many patients develop so severe allergy, that an indirect contact to horse is enough to release symptoms. Horse allergen extracts contain at least three different major allergens. Horse serum albumin is known to be an important allergen in epithelium extracts and allergic components have also been identified in horse dander preparations (101, 403, 418, 421, 423, 425, 426). Partial identity between antigens in horse serum and in extract of hair and dandruff of cow, dog, cat, guinea pig and in extract of house dust has been demonstrated (418).

Phadebas RAST®/Phadezym RAST® allergen e3 is acknowledged to be highly sensitive and specific (429).

Phadebas RAST®/Phadezym RAST® allergen e3 is produced by coupling an allergen extract of horse dander of high purity to activated paper discs. The content of allergens emanating from the desquamated epithelial cells is high while the serum protein concentration is low.

References: 101, 403, 418, 421, 423, 425, 426, 429

Further reading: 23, 347, 386, 391, 412, 415, 417, 430, 435, 437, 438

The sources of allergenic substances in cows are epithelia, dandruff, hair and milk. Some molecular fractions in cow hair have been identified as allergenic. Moreover, common antigens found in both cow's milk and cow hair have been isolated (347, 349, 351, 353, 373, 375, 376).

Allergy to cow has been reported in an allergic population with an incidence of 15 % (438). A comparison has been made, by measuring specific IgE in a group of allergic patients, between cow dander and cow serum coupled to allergen discs. Of 32 patient sera, 23 were positive to cow dander but only 2 were positive to cow serum and 30 patients were negative (158). Thus, those patients who had IgE antibodies to cow dander, also had antibodies to cow serum, but not the reverse.

ALLERGO-DISCS® for other domestic animal allergy testing are available for swine, sheep and goat epithelia, e83, e81 and e80, respectively.

Phadebas RAST®/Phadezym RAST® allergen e4 is acknowledged to be highly sensitive and specific (121, 386, 387).

Phadebas RAST®/Phadezym RAST® allergen e4 is produced by coupling an allergen extract of cow dander to activated paper discs.

References: 121, 158, 347, 349, 351, 353, 373, 375, 376, 386, 387, 438

Further reading: 335, 337, 345, 390, 391, 396, 444

e5 Dog dander

Dog allergens are described under the e2 disc, dog epithelium.

The e5 disc will detect dog sensitive patients with elevated concentrations of IgE-antibodies to

> dog-specific allergens from epithelia/dander

> the dander allergen shared by dog and cat

> animal serum proteins (due to cross-reactivity between dog and cat, possibly also to other animals such as horse, cow, rabbit).

> various combinations of these three allergen categories.

Phadebas RAST®/Phadezym RAST® allergen e5 is produced by coupling an allergen extract of a mixture of equal amount of Alsatian and poodle dander to activated paper discs.

Further reading: 385, 407

Guinea pig is widely used as a laboratory animal but increasingly also kept as a pet. Allergic reactions to laboratory animals is acknowledged. Components from epithelium have been recognized as highly allergenic as well as components excreted into the urine (375). A population of patients positive to Guinea pig epithelium (e6) were screened for raised specific IgE concentration against Hamster (e84), but only 9 out of 83 patients were positive (233). ALLERGO-DISCS® are available for other laboratory animals: mouse epithelia, urine proteins and serum proteins e71, e72, e76, respectively; rat epithelia, urine and serum proteins, e73, e74, e75; and rabbit and hamster epithelia e82 and e84, respectively.

Phadebas RAST®/Phadezym RAST® is acknowledged to be highly sensitive and specific (376).

Phadebas RAST®/Phadezym RAST® allergen e6 is produced by coupling an extract of Guinea pig epithelium to activated paper discs.

References: 233, 370, 375

Further reading: 335, 396, 404, 412, 417, 435

Pigeon is perhaps the first bird tamed by man. Figurines and mosaics portray the bird dating back to 4500 B.C. in Mesopotamia. The Egyptians included pigeon as an integral part of their diet.

Pigeon droppings are a ubiquitous urban allergen. The rock-pigeons lived in the craggy cliffs of southern Europe and were introduced to the New World. There they immediately adapted finding roosts behind billboards, in church steeples and public buildings with stone façades. Their droppings cause not only allergic reactions but other diseases as well.

'Bird fanciers' disease is one form of extrinsic allergic alveolitis disease (289). ALLERGO-DISCS® are available for testing for allergy to goose, budgerigar, chicken and duck feathers e71, e78, e85 and e86, respectively and also budgerigar droppings, e77 and serum proteins, e79.

Cross-reactivity among bird allergens has been reported (289, 294).

Phadebas RAST®/Phadezym RAST® allergen e7 is produced by coupling an allergen extract of sterilized pigeon droppings to activated paper discs.

References: 289, 294

House dust is a very heterogenic material, known as a cause of allergic rhinitis, conjunctivitis and bronchial asthma. It is a mixture of different allergenic compounds such as animal and human dander, moulds, mites and bacteria (43, 231, 315, 319, 443). Mites, *Dermatophagoides pteronyssinus* (d1) and *Dermatophagoides farinae* (d2), and Cockroach (i6) are regarded as the most important allergens (4, 69, 230, 235, 236, 298, 321). A specific house dust allergen has been suggested (215). However, this hypothesis has never been widely accepted.

Phadebas RAST®/Phadezym RAST® allergens h1-h4 are produced using different commercial sources. Each commercial extract contains its own spectrum of allergens, varying both in number and concentration.These discs, while not subject to Pharmacia's strict quality control, are made available for the convenience of those using the Phadebas RAST®/ Phadezym RAST® test system. The results indicated by Phadebas RAST®/ Phadezym RAST® allergens h1-h4 correspond to the different concentrations of antibodies directed to the individual allergens on the disc (229). The results aid in diagnosis as well as narrowing the field for further *in vitro* testing for animal epithelia, moulds, mites, cockroaches and other house dust components.

References: 4, 43, 69, 215, 229, 230, 231, 235, 236, 298, 315, 319, 321

Further reading: 23, 171, 172, 176, 204, 211, 212, 214, 221, 294.

Moulds and yeast

Moulds as inhalant allergens are of primary importance in seasonal allergic asthma and rhinitis. While there are some seasonal variations and certain peak periods most moulds have the capability of living year-round indoors as well as outdoors. *Cladosporium* can live under refrigeration and *Aspergillus* thrives at 40°C. Mould spores establish new colonies quickly making elimination difficult. From 4-30 % of atopic patients react to common mould allergens (322).

Fungal spores are more abundant than any other air-borne particles found in the atmosphere including pollen grains. They are also much smaller than pollen grains. Thus it is easier for the spores to be inhaled directly into the sensitive mucosa to cause asthma. One avoidance measure is to remain indoors on windy days after a first frost when spores are released in abundance. But, it is almost impossible to escape mould spores so prevalent in- and out-of-doors.

Very little is known about the antigenic and allergenic relations among the different fungi. However, several constituents have been characterized. A patient is seldomly allergic to only a single mould.

The raw material for the mould allergen discs has been carefully collected and purified to remove extraneous antigenic material. The moulds are grown on antigen-free substrates with the result being pure mould preparations.

Reference: 322

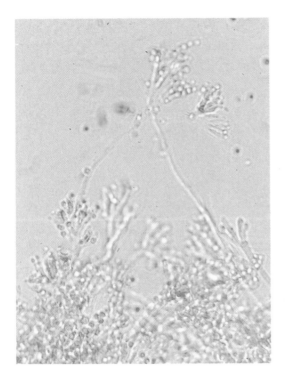

There are about 200 species of *Penicillium.* The contamination of a bacterial culture by a stray assexual spore of *P.notatum* and then the inhibition of bacterial growth led to Alexander Fleming's discovery of penicillin. Secondary metabolites from members of *Penicillium* have been revolutionary in combatting infectious diseases such as pneumonia and gonnorhoea. Two *Penicillium* strains are used in making blue and green mould cheese, *P.camenbertii* and *P.roquefortii.* An ALLERGO-DISCS® is available for mouldy cheese, f82.

Penicillium grows in dusty green colonies and dominates in temperate soils where spores are easily released into the atmosphere. Indoors it is the familiar blue-green mould found on stale bread, citrus fruits, apples and as a contaminant in rye flour in industrial bakeries.

Penicillium contrasts with most other moulds in that it has no big seasonal variations but reaches peak concentration in the winter and spring. It is a major cause of indoor mould allergy.

Phadebas RAST®/Phadezym RAST® allergen m1 is acknowledged to be highly sensitive and specific (4, 80, 328).

Phadebas RAST®/Phadezym RAST® allergen m1 is produced by coupling an allergen extract of spores and mycelia of *Penicillium notatum* to activated paper discs.

References: 4, 80, 328

Further reading: 130

The genus *Cladosporium* with its 25 different species has the widest distribution of all moulds throughout the world, especially in temperate regions. It is the dominant air-borne mould in many areas. It is a secondary invader of leaves on trees in the autumn and can be liberated by raindrops, mists or wind. The colonies are a velvety olive green or shades of brown or greenish-grey.

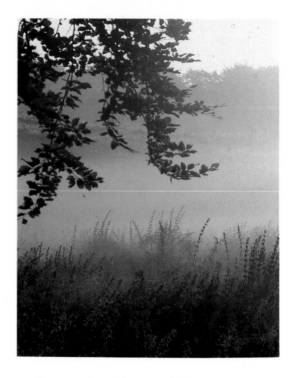

Some *Cladosporium* species can grow below 20°C which makes it a serious problem for refrigerated foods. It is often found in houses with poor ventilation or around moist window frames where it covers the entire painted area. Also it is found in houses with thatched rooves, or those in low damp environments. The mould frequently causes blackening of cereal ears. *Cladosporium* has also been isolated from fuel tanks causing problems for the petrol industry and has been found in some face creams, paints, soil and textiles.

The complex antigens and allergens in *Cladosporium herbarum* have been characterized (323, 324, 326). *Cladosporium* is regarded as the primary source of mould allergy.

Phadebas RAST®/Phadezym RAST® allergen m2 is acknowledged to be highly sensitive and specific (4, 328).

Phadebas RAST®/Phadezym RAST® allergen m2 is produced by coupling an allergen extract of spores and mycelia of *Cladosporium herbarum* to activated paper discs.

References : 4, 323, 324, 326, 328

Further reading: 98, 305, 310, 311, 313, 315, 319, 321, 322, 443

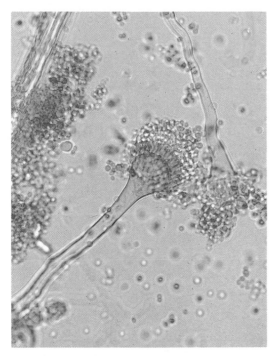

Aspergillus fumigatus is found in fertile soil, decaying vegetable matter, flours, swimming pool water but is most commonly cultured from houses, basements, bedding, house dust and raw textile materials. A non-toxic *Aspergillus* strain is used in making vinegar and soy sauce. *Aspergillus* thrives at 40°C whereas most other moulds require more moderate temperatures. The spores are at peak concentrations in the autumn and winter when patients begin to experience symptoms.

The spores are inhaled and deposited in the sensitive mucosa. Inhalation of the spores can lead to several diseases the severity of which depends on the host's immune response: Allergic asthma, Aspergilloma (fungus ball), hypersensitivity pneumonitis, invasive aspergillosis and allergic bronchopulmonary aspergillosis (ABPA). Aspergilloma usually affects non-atopics who develop a fungal ball in the lungs, have a chronic cough and can be misdiagnosed as having tuberculosis.

Allergic bronchopulmonary aspergillosis is almost always atopic and the patients have had bronchial asthma at one time. It can take young asthmatics 25 years or more to develop ABPA but only 3 to 5 years for patients who develop asthma after age 30.

Serum IgE as well as IgG antibodies have been measured during the course of these diseases (289, 300, 301). The elevated total IgE and IgG antibodies provide useful serological aids in diagnosis where other clinical and laboratory manifestations are not unique to ABPA (294). Cross-reactivity among the different *Aspergillus* species is assumed but unique antigens have been identified (298). Phadebas RAST®/Phadezym RAST® allergen m3 is acknowledged to be highly sensitive and specific (328).

References: 289, 298, 300, 301, 328

Further reading: 239, 260, 263, 271, 273, 276, 277, 282, 287, 315, 319, 321, 322, 391

Mucor is called a "sugar fungus" because it attacks carbohydrates. It can be found on rotting vegetable material such as mushrooms, horse dung and soils. In the household it grows in soft fruits, sour milk and marmelade. It is the dominant mould in floor dust. The mould helps break down fruit pectins and so is used in fruit pulp and juice production.

Mucor racemosus requires a 92 % humidity to grow and 95 % humidity for sporulation. It is considered an indoor mould thus influencing perennial asthma and rhinitis.

Phadebas RAST®/Phadezym RAST® allergen m4 is acknowledged to be highly sensitive and specific (328).

Phadebas RAST®/Phadezym RAST® allergen m4 is produced by coupling an allergen extract of spores and mycelia of *Mucor racemosus* to activated paper discs.

References: 328

Further reading: 4, 98, 315, 319, 321

Candida albicans is a dimorphic fungus which means it grows as a yeast in a carbohydrate-rich medium but starts forming hyphae when the medium is low in nutrients.

Candida is commonly present in man, but rarely causes severe infections.

The role of *Candida* as a cause of allergy has been much disputed. Positive skin reactions are frequently obtained in patients without clinical evidence of *Candida* infection or allergic disease (141, 151). In a population of 1300 asthmatic children, 5% had positive skin prick test results to *Candida albicans* (139). Phadebas RAST®/Phadezym RAST® allergen m5 is acknowledged to be highly sensitive and specific (152, 154).

Phadebas RAST®/Phadezym RAST® allergen m5 is produced by coupling an allergen extract of disrupted cells of *Candida albicans* to activated paper discs.

References: 139, 141, 151, 152, 154

Further reading: 163, 164, 169, 288

Alternaria species occur world-wide and are considered outdoor moulds. As such, *Alternaria* follows a seasonal pattern appearing when the weather is warm and humid. *Alternaria* is found on fruits and textiles. Black spots on tomatoes may be caused by *Alternaria.* Spores are thought to have a connection to Baker's asthma. Species of the genus *Alternaria* have been found to contain major allergens (238, 240, 243, 253, 257).

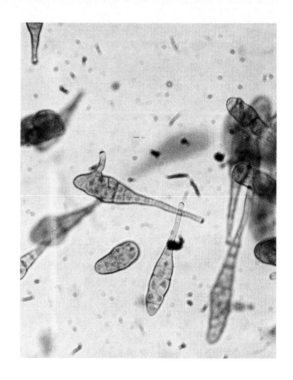

Phadebas RAST®/Phadezym RAST® allergen m6 is acknowledged to be highly sensitive and specific (80, 395, 328).

Phadebas RAST®/Phadezym RAST ® allergen m6 is produced by coupling an allergen extract of spores and mycelia of *Alternaria alternata* to activated paper discs.

References: 80, 238, 240, 243, 253, 257, 328, 395

Further reading: 4, 43, 69, 298, 315, 443

Mites

Most allergology researchers of today agree that mites are the most important allergen source in house dust. As early as 1928 the presence of mites in house dust was known (227). In 1964 this finding was reaffirmed and enlarged upon when *Dermatophagoides pteronyssinus* and *Dermatophagoides farinae* were identified in house dust samples from all over the world (222, 225, 226).

The geographical distribution of these two species does not differ significantly, but the relative frequency does. *D.pteronyssinus* dominates most of Europe and Great Britain. *D.farinae* is an important allergen in North America and Japan, and also common in parts of Italy and Turkey. In the Far East both species are equally prevalent. Altitude plays a role because low damp areas with high humidity are preferable. Allergenic mite sources are almost impossible to get rid of. Killing living mites with pesticides merely results in dead mites, also a potent allergen source. In addition, mite faeces have been shown to be highly allergenic (76).

Besides discs for *D.pteronyssinus* and *D.farinae,* there are ALLERGO-DISCS® available for testing storage mite allergy, *Acarus siro* (d70), *Lepidoglyphus destructor* (d71), *Tyrophagus putrescentiae* (d72), and *Glycyphagus domesticus* (d73).

Common symptoms in mite allergy are perennial type asthma, rhinitis and conjunctivitis, often with nocturnal or early morning episodes.

References: 76, 222, 225, 226, 227

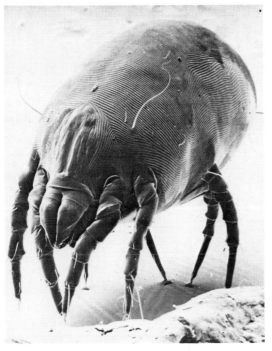

Mites have a life-cycle of about 2 to 3½ months. They live in house dust and thrive in high humidity. Upholstered furniture, mattresses and carpeting are natural habitats for mites. They perform a service by feeding on other unwanted components in house dust as well as human and animal dander.

D.pteronyssinus dominates most of Europe and Great Britain.

D.pteronyssinus and *D.farinae* have about 11 and 7 allergens, respectively, some of which they have in common. However, there are also antigens unique to each species (339).

Phadebas RAST®/Phadezym RAST® allergen d1 is acknowledged to be highly sensitive and specific (23, 130, 215, 219).

Phadebas RAST®/Phadezym RAST® allergen d1 is produced by coupling an allergen extract of *Dermatophagoides pteronyssinus* to activated paper discs.

References: 23,130,215,219,339

Further reading: 207, 209, 210

Dermatophagoides farinae has many of the same characteristics as *D.pteronyssinus.* It has been suggested that mite sensitivity in asthmatic children can be correlated to which part of the year they were born. The mite sensitive children were characteristically born during the autumn or winter and tended to develop asthma before five years (226).

The prevalence of allergic reactions to the mite species *Dermatophagoides farinae* is shown to be extremely high in North America and Japan. However, large numbers of this species have also been found in parts of Italy and Turkey, and in the Far East.

D.pteronyssinus and *D.farinae* have about 11 and 7 allergens, respectively, some of which they have in common (339). However, there are also antigens unique to each species.

Phadebas RAST®/Phadezym RAST® allergen d2 is acknowledged to be highly sensitive and specific (80).

Phadebas RAST®/Phadezym RAST® allergen d2 is produced by coupling an allergen extract of *Dermatophagoides farinae* to activated paper discs.

References: 80, 226, 339

Venoms

Insect sting allergy is not a very common form of allergy, though it can be life-threatening (122, 124, 127, 130). It is probably the oldest documented form of allergy. The absolute incidence of this type of allergy in different countries is not known. In North America, however, the incidence has been calculated to 0.5-0.8 % of the population. In the United States, bees kill more people than snakes, and *Vespidae* are the third most deadly venomous animal. Death usually comes within the first hour after a sting and is attributed to insect allergy and not the toxic effect of the venom. It is thought that heat stroke or heart attack may be given as a cause of death when actually it was the result of a sting. The severity of the reaction depends on the amount of venom injected and its components. *Vespidae* stings often cause secondary infections because of the scavenger nature of these insects and higher risk of bacterial contamination. An ALLERGO-DISCS® for Fire ant, a member of the *Hymenoptera* venoms *Solenopsis ivicta,* i70, is also available.

The taxonomic relationship of some *Hymenoptera* species is outlined in the diagram. Different colloquial names are used for the same species throughout the world. A sampling of some names for 'wasp' and 'hornet' is included p. IX:3. In the text, the common English is given along with Latin.

Vespidae were introduced in Australia and New Zealand by accident. Because of the mild winters, they have become a problem especially in New Zealand where they live two to three years and become very large and aggressive. In the autumn they eat rotten, fermenting fruit and become intoxicated and even more fierce.

Vespula threatens the major fruit growing areas in New Zealand where they have killed great numbers of Honey bees, thereby reducing pollination.

Vespula species prefer cooler climates whereas *Polistes* are more common in warmer parts of the world. *Apis mellifera,* prized for its honey and pollination activities, has been spread throughout most of the world.

Traditional extracts for diagnosis and treatment of insect sting allergy were made from the whole bodies of the animals. In recent years, venom of bees and wasps have been shown to be superior compared to whole body extracts (25, 112, 114, 117, 131, 135). Venoms are collected through electric stimulation (Honey bee) or manual dissection of the venom sac (wasps and hornets) (100). Most studies generally indicate that honey bee and vespid venoms possess different antigenic properties. Within the group

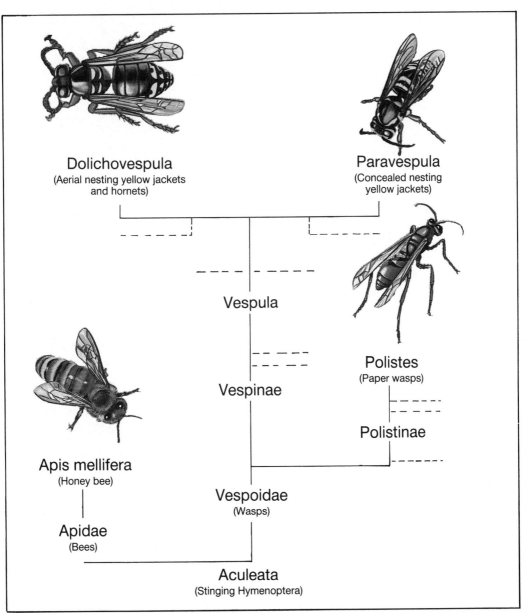

Dolichovespula
(Aerial nesting yellow jackets and hornets)

Paravespula
(Concealed nesting yellow jackets)

Vespula

Polistes
(Paper wasps)

Vespinae

Polistinae

Apis mellifera
(Honey bee)

Apidae
(Bees)

Vespoidae
(Wasps)

Aculeata
(Stinging Hymenoptera)

of vespid venoms there appears to be both cross-reacting and distinctive antigens (92, 96,325).

References: 25, 92, 96, 100, 112, 114, 117, 122, 124, 127, 130, 131, 135, 325

Further reading: 177, 186, 187, 290

The natural range of the Honey bee is thought to be Africa, Europe and the Middle East for *A.mellifera* and Japan, India and Indochina for *A.cerona.* Now, Honey bees have been domesticated and spread throughout the world. In Canada, bee-keepers even take advantage of the lush blooming of spring wild flowers in the far north by flying their bee colonies into the wilderness thus increasing the honey yield. Most Honey bee stings occur in bee-keepers and their families or in people who walk barefoot on lawns containing clover. Honey bee is the only stinging *Hymenoptera* that nearly always leaves the stinger in the skin of the victim.

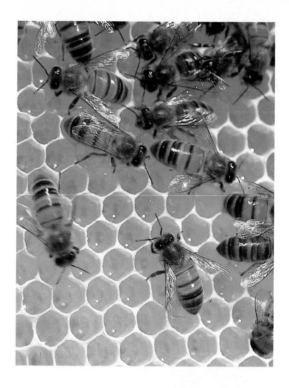

Different major compounds of bee venom have been extensively studied (1, 30, 32, 35, 38, 52, 67, 440). The venom contains several components of a protein nature virtually all of which are allergenic, especially hyluronidase and phospholipase A which have shown reactivity to IgE antibodies from almost all patients with insect sting allergy. There is no cross-reactivity between honey bee venom and the major venom of the *Vespidae,* called antigen 5 (30).

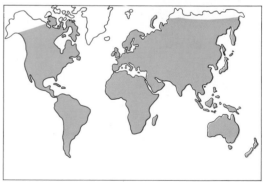

Phadebas RAST®/Phadezym RAST® allergen i1 is acknowledged to be highly sensitive and specific (86, 88, 90, 115, 165, 173).

Phadebas RAST®/Phadezym RAST® allergen i1 is produced by coupling Honey bee venom, obtained through electric stimulation of bees, to activated paper discs.

References: 1, 30, 32, 35, 38, 52, 67, 86, 88, 90, 115, 165, 173, 440

The White-faced hornets live in large colonies with 50 to 2000 individuals. They often build their nests on or around human dwellings. Stinging incidents often occur when man accidentally disturbs a nest while engaged in yardwork or house repairs. White-faced hornet is rare in Europe, however of great importance on the North American continent.

An extensive cross-reactivity has been shown to other wasp species (177, 325).

Phadebas RAST®/Phadezym RAST® allergen i2 is produced by coupling venom from dissected venom sacs from White-faced hornet to activated paper discs.

References: 177, 325

SOCIAL WASPS
THE WORDS 'WASP' AND 'HORNET' IN 32 LANGUAGES

	WASP	HORNET
American	yellow jacket	hornet
Arabic	dabbour	dabbour
Bulgarian	ocá	–
Chinese	wong fong	tai wong fong
Czech	vosa	srsen
Danish	hveps	gedehams
Dutch	wesp	hoornaar
Farsi	zanbour	zanbour-e-sorkh or, zanbour-e-dorosht
Finnish	ampiainen	herhiläinen
French	guêpe	frelon
Gaelic	connspeach	connsbeach
German	wespe	hornisse
Greek	sphex	meg-al-ee sphex
Hebrew	tzir-ah daboor	–
Hindi	tatsiya	hara
Hungarian	daraźs	lodaraze
Irish	eirkveach	–
Italian	vespa	calabrone
Japanese	–	suzume-bah-chi
Latin	vespula	vespa
Malay	pěnyěngat	tebuan
Norwegian	veps	gjetehams or, geitehams
Polish	osa	szerszeń
Portugese	vespa	vespão
Romanian	viespe	gărgăun
Russian	oca	chershyen
Serbocroat	osa	stršen
Slovene	osa	sršen
Spanish	avispa	moscardón or, crabrón
Swedish	geting	bålgeting
Turkish	esek arisi	büyük esek arisi
Welsh	gwenynen	cacynen

Among the *Vespula* species, *Vespula vulgaris* is the group of Yellow jackets which is responsible for inflicting the greatest proportion of stings. They live in large colonies, with 500-5000 individuals (325). When a colony is disturbed, the sentry wasps fly out, find the intruder and begin to sting. The venom contains an alarm substance which tells the other wasps the location of the first sting. Then they continue stinging around that site.

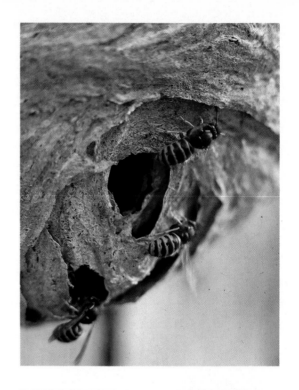

New colonies are initiated by a single queen who has survived the winter. Later in the season, the worker wasps are more likely to sting when the colony begins to decline. *Vespula* species thrives in cooler climates in the north temperate zone and in Australia, South Africa and Chile.

Different major allergens from Yellow jacket venom have been isolated (58, 62, 73, 78, 110, 189) and cross-reactivities between components of venoms from different wasp species have been identified (92, 96). Thus, elevated levels of IgE antibodies with affinity

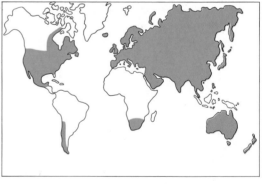

to Yellow jacket venom could be measured in patients sensitized to the European wasp as well as in patients sensitized with the American species, Yellow jacket.

Phadebas RAST®/Phadezym RAST® allergen i3 is acknowledged to be highly sensitive and specific (137, 136, 165, 356).

Phadebas RAST®/Phadezym RAST® allergen i3 is produced by coupling venom from dissected sacs from *Vespula* species to activated paper discs.

References: 58, 62, 73, 78, 92, 96, 110, 136, 137, 165, 189, 325, 356

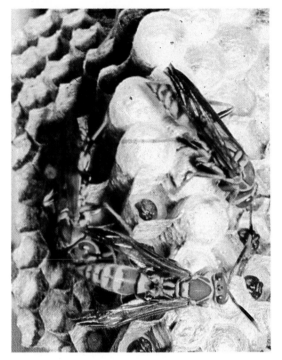

Paper wasps build single comb nests above the ground, often attaching them to buildings, so man often accidentally comes in contact with these insects. The colonies are relatively small, 10-250 individuals. Only fertilized queens overwinter and a new nest is begun by one queen.

Drawings found on the tombs of Egyptian Pharaohs are similar to *Polistes.* Aristophanes, the Greek dramatist, wrote a play, ''The Wasps'' thus clothing the word 'wasp' with the meaning it still has today - 'spiteful'. In Jamaica, coconut pollination is carried out by wasps in addition to bees.

Paper wasps are frequently found in North America as well as in Europe. Cross-reactivity patterns to other wasp species are not as thoroughly documented as those among *Vespidae* (92, 179, 189).

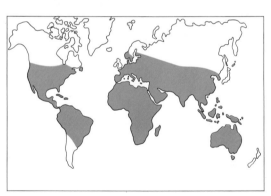

Phadebas RAST®/Phadezym RAST® allergen i4 is acknowledged to be highly sensitive and specific (136).

Phadebas RAST®/Phadezym RAST® allergen i4 is produced by coupling venom from dissected sacs from *Polistes* species to activated paper discs.

References: 92, 136, 179, 189

Yellow hornet, as well as the White-faced hornet, build rather large nests, often hanging from branches or on eaves of houses. In general, they sting only when their nest is disturbed.

Most Yellow hornets are found in the near Artic regions in Asia, Europe and North America. They were introduced in Australia.

Yellow hornet has been shown to cross-react to a very high degree with White-faced hornet (177, 189).

Pha debas RAST®/Phadezym RAST® allergen i5 is produced by coupling venom from dissected sacs from *Dolichovespula arenaria* to activated paper discs.

References: 177, 189

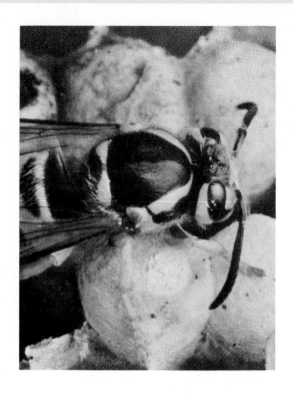

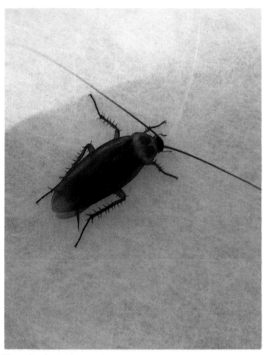

Tropical cockroach

Cockroaches eat almost everything from household refuse to drainpipe waste and other insects. For every cockroach that is seen, twenty may be waiting for darkness to become active. Breeding takes place in kitchens, bathrooms or near the boiler of the central heating system. Radio and television sets may become infested, as well as the insulation of refrigerators and sometimes ovens. *B.germanica* is a cosmopolitan cockroach.

Hypersensitivity to cockroach allergens has been frequently reported during recent years and cockroach hypersensitivity has even been suggested to be as prevalent as ragweed hypersensitivity in the US (150). Cockroach antigens cause immediate skin reactions and immediate bronchoconstriction. Cockroach allergens have been identified as a potent allergen source in house dust (150, 153). Major cockroach allergens have been isolated (140, 142).

Phadebas RAST®/Phadezym RAST® allergen i6 is acknowledged to be highly sensitive and specific (24).

Phadebas RAST®/Phadezym RAST® allergen i6 is produced by coupling a whole body extract of *Blatella germanica* to activated paper discs.

References: 24, 140, 142 , 150, 153

Further reading: 156

Drugs

Drug allergens are small molecules and in order to provoke the immune system they have to combine with proteins. Such complexes are spontaneously formed in the body (178).

Therapeutic penicillin is the most common cause of hypersensitivity reactions to drug treatment. However, only a few of them seem to be truly allergic in nature. Estimates of the incidence of adverse reactions range from 1 to 10 % in patients receiving this medication (205). The number of true allergic reactions is certainly lower (188, 202).

The penicilloyl residue is considered to be the major allergenic penicillin determinant (188). Minor determinants might be present to a limited extent (188, 202), and severe reactions to them may sometimes occur.

Most common immediate type allergic reactions are urticaria and various skin rashes (185).

Compared to *in vivo* tests used for diagnosis of sensitivity to penicillin, *in vitro* determination of specific IgE antibodies is safe and convenient (175). Phadebas RAST® allergens c1 and c2 measure specific IgE antibodies to the major allergenic determinants of therapeutic penicillin.

References: 175, 178, 185, 188, 202, 205

A number of commercially available penicillins have the chemical structure (6-aminopenicillanic acid) required for being considered as a potential precursor of penicilloyl. Penicilloyl G is derived from Benzyl penicillin. Direct correlations have been found between levels of IgE antibody specific to this antigen, measured by the RAST-technique, and findings from *in vivo* tests (170, 166, 162).

Phadebas RAST® allergen c1 is acknowledged to be highly sensitive and specific (138, 306, 312, 320).

Phadebas RAST® allergen c1 is produced by coupling a conjugate of Benzyl penicilloyl and human serum albumin to activated paper discs.

References: 138, 162, 166, 170, 306, 312, 320

A number of commercially available penicillins have the chemical structure (6-aminopenicillanic acid) required for being considered as a potential precursor of penicilloyl. Penicilloyl V is derived from Phenoxy-methyl penicillin. Direct correlations have been found between levels of IgE antibody specific to this antigen, measured by the RAST-technique, and findings from *in vivo* tests (162, 166, 170).

Phadebas RAST® allergen c2 is acknowledged to be highly sensitive and specific (138, 306, 312, 320).

Phadebas RAST® allergen c2 is produced by coupling a conjugate of Phenoxy-methyl penicilloyl and human serum albumin to activated paper discs.

References: 138, 162, 166, 170, 306, 312, 320

Parasites

The clinical manifestations of parasitic diseases are so general that diagnosis based on symptomology is nearly impossible. The helminths especially produce indefinite symptoms.

For decades diagnosis of parasitic infection has been carried out by traditional methods, e.g. by searching for egg or worms in faeces. Diagnostic laboratory techniques such as hemagglutination, immuno-fluorescence and flocculation tests have been used.

Diagnosis is especially difficult in non-endemic areas where clinicians have less experience with parasite infection and patients can be misdiagnosed. Incidence of parasitic infection in non-endemic areas is rising because of increased travel.

Many parasitic infections will cause substantially raised total IgE. Levels up to 10-20 000 kU/L, have been measured by Phadebas IgE PRIST® or Phadezym IgE PRIST®. Specific IgE antibodies to parasites have been found in connection with infections due to *Echinococcus, Ascaris* and *Schistosoma.* The behaviour characteristics of the parasites may determine whether there will be raised IgE levels. Helminths restricted to the lumen of the digestive tract do not appear to have raised IgE levels (83).

Specific diagnosis of the offending parasite can be achieved by using Phadebas RAST®/Phadezym RAST® allergens p1-p3 for parasite IgE antibodies detection. Measurement of IgE antibodies has been shown to be more specific for parasite diagnosis than measurement of IgG and other antibodies (280, 334).

References: 83, 280, 334

The adult worms usually live in the small intestine and live on partially digested food of the host. The eggs are passed in the faeces, form larvae in the soil and become infective. Temperatures lower than 25°C inhibit growth. Once in the body of the host, they eventually arrive in the intestine where they live for about 12-18 months.

Children are more likely to be infected because of increased exposure to contaminated soils transmitted hand-to-mouth. Symptoms include allergic reactions, asthmatic attacks and oedema of the lips. The high incidence of allergic asthma and increased IgE-mediated skin activity in South Africa has been associated with *Ascaris* (75).

Ascaris is a prominent parasite in both temperate and tropical zones but most common in warm countries, especially where the sanitation is poor. It is thought that about 900 million people are infected with the parasite. In lands where 'night soil' is a common fertilizer, people of all ages can become infected from vegetables.

Raised levels of IgE antibody against *Ascaris* have been reported (75, 295, 399). Cross-reactivity with other nematodes such as *Toxocara* and *Filaria* could be expected.

Phadebas RAST®/Phadezym RAST® p1 is acknowledged to be highly sensitive and specific (280).

Phadebas RAST®/Phadezym RAST® p1 is produced by coupling an extract of adult *Ascaris suum* worms from swine to activated paper discs.

References: 75, 280, 295, 399

When the egg of *Echinococcus granulosus* is ingested by man, it is carried to different parts of the body by the blood stream. Cysts develop much like slow-growing tumours. They are found on the liver, in the lungs and abdomen and other organs. If a cyst erupts, allergic symptoms such as urticaria follow. If a great deal of hydatid material is released into the blood stream, anaphylactic symptoms and even sudden death may occur. Hydatid cysts may be mistaken for tubercullosis, syphillus, various malignancies and hepatic cirrhosis.

The incidence of infection is high in sheep-grazing areas where association with dogs is intimate such as in Australia, New Zealand and the Middle East. In Canada and Alaska, moose and caribou are the intermediate hosts and the wolf is the definitive host. Infection often takes place in childhood but the parasite can easily be transmitted to man from the fur of infected animals or animals who have rolled in infected faeces.

E.granulosus is found in the Middle East, Oceania, Southeast Asia, and parts of Africa and South America. *E.multilocularis* is carried in cats and foxes and is found in Russia, Siberia, Alaska and occasionally the midwestern US.

In a study conducted in Germany, 11 out of 13 patients with *E.multilocularis* were detected with the p2 disc (125). In another group of 107 infected patients, the p2 disc detected both *E.granulosus* and *E.multilocularis* in 99 % (126). The p2 disc has been shown to be very useful and as good as the traditional immunological methods for diagnosis (389). The Casoni test for hydatid parasites may show as high as 18 % false positives (338). In Mexico, a group of patients with cerebral cysticercosis (caused by *Taenia solium's* larval stage) were 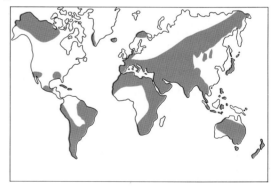 screened with the p2 disc. All were negative which suggests an absence of cross-reactivity even though *T.solium* and *E.granulosus* are related (197).

Phadebas RAST®/Phadezym RAST® p2 is acknowledged to be highly sensitive and specific (79, 111, 125, 126).

Phadebas RAST®/Phadezym RAST® p2 is produced by coupling *Echinococcus granulosus* hydatid cyst fluid of human origin to activated paper discs.

References: 79, 111, 125, 126, 197, 338, 389

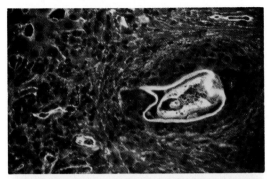

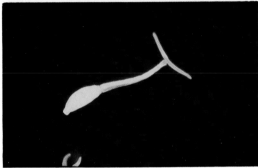

Schistosoma egg *Schistosoma cercarie*

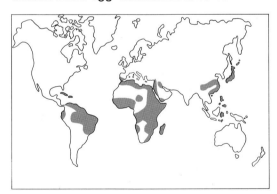

The *Schistosoma* egg is carried in fresh water snails. The *cercariae* begin the incubation period when they penetrate the skin of man and may induce a rash. The immature worms then invade the liver and other organs. Toxic and allergic reactions may cause urticaria, oedema, asthmatic attacks, leukocytis and eosinophilia. In light infections, the chronic disease begins after 4-5 years; in serious cases, after 1-2 years.

Shistosoma mansoni is commonly found in Arabia and Yemen, in the Nile Delta, central Africa, the northern and eastern regions of South America and the Caribbean Islands. The parasite was probably introduced in the New World by the slave trade. About 200 million people are infected.

S.haematobium is found in the Nile valley, most of Africa, Japan and the Middle East. *S.japonicum* is confined to the Far East.

In different studies, specific IgE antibodies against *Schistosoma* allergens have been identified (334, 336). In one study, patients known to be infected with *S.haematobium* were tested with the p3 discs. About 90 % were positive which indicates a high degree of cross-reactivity between the two species (26). In another study, 68 % of a patient group infected with *Schistosoma japonicum* were positive with the p3 disc, showing cross-reactivity also between *S.mansoni* and *S.japonicum* (53).

Phadebas RAST®/Phadezym RAST® p3 is acknowledged to be highly sensitive and specific (26, 53, 60).

Phadebas RAST®/Phadezym RAST® p3 is produced by coupling an extract of adult *Schistosoma mansoni* worms to activated paper discs.

References: 26, 53, 60, 334, 336

ALLERGO-DISCS®

ALLERGO-DISCS® are included as a separate chapter as they are produced by MIAB AB, under licence from Pharmacia. The discs have been selected to complement the range of Phadebas RAST®/Phadezym RAST® allergen preparations.

A separate reference list follows immediately after the chapter.

Pollens

g70 Elymus triticoides, Wild rye
g71 Phalaris arundinacea, Canary grass
t70 Morus alba, Mulberry

Foods

f76 Alpha-lactalbumin
f77 Beta-lactoglobulin
k78 Casein
f81 Cheese, Cheddar-type
f82 Cheese, mould type
f75 Egg yolk
f83 Chicken
f79 Gluten
f80 Lobster
f88 Mutton
f84 Kiwi fruit
f85 Celery
f86 Parsley
f87 Melons
f89 Mustard

Animal allergens

e88 Mouse
e71 Mouse epithelia
e72 Mouse urine proteins
e76 Mouse serum proteins
e87 Rat
e73 Rat epithelia
e74 Rat urine proteins
e75 Rat serum proteins
e80 Goat epithelia
e81 Sheep epithelia
e82 Rabbit epithelia
e83 Swine epithelia
e84 Hamster epithelia
e70 Goose feathers
e85 Chicken feathers
e86 Duck feathers
e78 Budgerigar feathers
e77 Budgerigar droppings
e79 Budgerigar serum proteins

Occupational allergens
Protein allergens

k70 Green coffee bean
k71 Castor bean
k72 Ispaghula
k73 Silk waste
k74 Silk

Chemical allergens

k75 TDI, toluene diisocyanate
k76 MDI, methylene diphenyl diisocyanate
k77 HDI, hexamethylene diisocyanate
k78 Ethylene oxide
k79 Phthalic anhydride

Mites

d70 Acarus siro
d71 Lepidoglyphus destructor
d72 Tyrophagus putrescentiae
d73 Glycyphagus domesticus

Venoms and insects

i70 Solenopsis invicta, Fire ant
i71 Aedes communis, Common mosquito
i72 Cladotanytarsus Lewisi, Green nimitti
i73 Chironomus Thummi Th, Blood worm

Drugs

c70 Insulin, porcine
c71 Insulin, bovine
c73 Insulin, human

Miscellaneous

o70 Seminal fluid

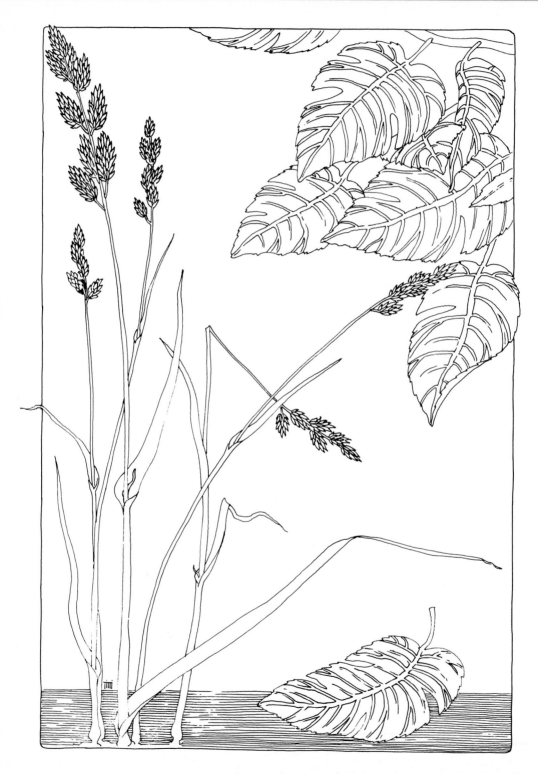

g70 *Elymus triticoides*
Wild rye grass

This is a pantemperate tribe notable for its cereal genera, wheat, barley and rye. The close relation speaks in favour of common cross-reactivity between *E.triticoides* and the cereals mentioned as well as with *E.arenarius*. It is widely distributed in the western US, from central Washington to Baja California, eastwards to Montana and New Mexico. It grows on river flats, saline meadows, sand-dunes and sage-brush deserts. In Europe the lyme-grass, *E.arenarius*, is common in the sand-dunes along the coasts. The pollen season is from June to August.

The pollen batch used for coupling to the discs has been found to be pure with less than 0.5 % detectable foreign pollens. See also Phadebas RAST®/ Phadezym RAST® allergen disc g5, Rye-grass.

g71 *Phalaris arundinacea*
Canary grass

The grass is widely distributed in the US with the exception of the most southern parts and it is rather common in Europe. It grows along river flats and coasts.

The pollen season is from June to August.

The pollen preparations used for coupling to the discs are of high quality with less than 0.5 % detectable contaminating foreign pollens.

t70 *Morus alba*
Mulberry

Morus alba, or the white mulberry tree, is a member of the family *Moraceae*. Other members include figs (*Ficus elastica*), bread-fruit (*Artocarpus*) and the American tropical rubber-tree (*Castilla elastica*). *M.alba* is a native of China but is now common in the eastern and midwestern USA.

Other species of the same family are red mulberry, black mulberry and Texas mulberry. Mulberries are popular for street planting for example in southern California and as ornamentals in the eastern US and in Europe (1). In some countries it is extensively cultivated along road sides, agricultural fields and in gardens. In Japan, mulberry leaves are fed to silkworms. It is wind-pollinated and is a dominating pollen in its region. The pollens are highly allergenic.

When studying the diurnal pollen periodicity, *Morus* shows an early morning pattern (2).

It can be assumed that *M.alba* to varying degrees cross-reacts with other species of the same family and cross-reactivity cannot be excluded with the elm family, *Ulmacea*. (See also Phadebas RAST®/Phadezym RAST® allergen disc t8, Elm). Furthermore, it is very likely that *M.alba* to a high degree cross-reacts with *Broussonetia papyrifera* (Paper mulberry) (3).

The pollen batch used for coupling to the discs has been found to be pure with less than 1 % detectable foreign pollens.

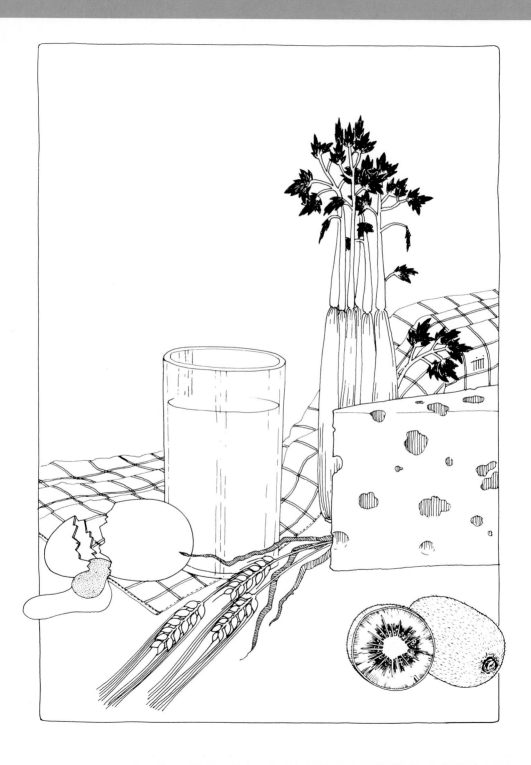

f76 Alpha-lactalbumin

Alpha-lactalbumin is regarded as one of the major cow's milk allergens. Cross-reactivity with the other bovine milk fractions has rarely been observed.

The allergenic material on the discs consists of pure alpha-lactalbumin isolated from cow's milk. See also Phadebas RAST®/Phadezym RAST® allergen disc f2, Whole milk.

f77 Beta-lactoglobulin

Beta-lactoglobulin is a bovine milk fraction which together with alpha-lactalbumin is regarded as one of the major allergens in cow's milk. Cross-reactivity with the other bovine milk fractions has rarely been observed.

The allergenic material consists of pure beta-lactoglobulin isolated from cow's milk.

f78 Casein

Together with alpha-lactalbumin and beta-lactoglobulin, casein is regarded as a major cow's milk allergen. Cross-reactivity with the other bovine milk fractions have rarely been observed.

The allergenic material consists of pure casein isolated from cow's milk.

f81 Cheese, Cheddar-type

The allergenic material consists of a mixture of processed and unprocessed cheese of the Cheddar-type. The discs contain some allergens present in cow's milk but there is no significant correlation with the ALLERGO-DISCS® cow's milk proteins.

f82 Cheese, mould-type

The allergenic material on the discs consists of a mixture of white mould cheese (Camembert and Brie) and green mould cheese (Gorgonzola and Roquefort). The discs contain some allergens present in cow's milk, but there is no significant correlation with the ALLERGO-DISCS® cow's milk proteins. Generally, sera from patients allergic to inhaled mould spores (*Aspergillus, Alternaria, Cladosporium* and *Penicillium*) do not react with these discs.

f75 Egg yolk

Egg allergy is considered to be less common than milk allergy but the allergic threshold is much lower. If a patient is egg-allergic, it doesn't matter if it is chicken, goose, duck or turkey; all eggs can produce symptoms. Egg or egg components are often used in the food industry and many foods have been prepared with egg or contain egg products. Some vaccines are cultured on egg embryos as well.

The egg yolk has been found to contain proteins wholly or closely related to all the allergens in egg white, although the amount of many of these proteins is probably small. Several proteins cross-reacting between egg yolk and hen/chicken sera and skin have been demonstrated (4).

The allergenic material on the discs consists of unfractionated egg yolk from fresh white leghorn egg. See also Phadebas RAST®/Phadezym RAST® allergen disc f1, Egg white.

f83 Chicken

Chicken meat belongs to the group of foods that rather often elicits allergic symptoms. The allergens in the meat seem to be different from the major allergens in hen's egg. However, cross-reactivity may probably be found within the poultry group such as turkey, goose and squab. The allergenic material on the discs consists of fresh chicken meat. No contaminating fish-protein material or antibiotics such as penicillin have been detected.

Gluten is the elastic rubbery protein in wheat, rye, oat and barley that binds the dough in foods such as bread, biscuits, cakes and pastry. Gliadin, a component in gluten, has been shown to elicit IgE-mediated allergic reactions and patients extremely allergic to gliadin have been described (5). Patients with gluten intolerance (celiac disease) are usually weakly positive or negative in RAST to gluten. Elevated total IgE levels have been reported and may be a consistent finding in celiac disease (6). Hypersensitivity to gluten requires avoiding wheat and rye, possibly also barley and oats.

The allergenic material on the discs consists of gliadin prepared from wheat. See also Phadebas RAST®/Phadezym RAST cereal discs, f4, f5, f6, f7, f11, wheat, rye, barley, oats and buckwheat, respectively.

Allergy to crustaceans such as lobster, crab and shrimps can cause severe reactions such as anaphylaxis in the highly susceptible individual. These reactions are mainly IgE-mediated.

Results from immunological studies suggest that there are cross-reacting allergens within the class *Crustacea* which have the potential to sensitize individuals to other members prior to exposure. See also Phadebas RAST®/ Phadezym RAST® allergen discs f23, Crab and f24, Shrimp.

The allergenic material coupled to the discs consists of boiled, frozen Canadian lobster meat.

It cannot be excluded that mutton has some allergens in common with sheep's wool. Mutton is regarded as a weak allergen and positive reactions are only seen in extreme food allergic patients. The allergenic material on the discs consists of fresh mutton. No contaminating meat tenderizer such as papain has been detected on the discs.

f84 Kiwi fruit

Kiwi fruit has been reported to cause allergic symptoms in highly sensitive patients (7). Pollen-allergic individuals seem to be prone to develop allergy to kiwi fruit.

The allergenic material on the discs consists of pulp from the Kiwi fruit (Chinese gooseberry, *Actinidia chinensis*).

f85 Celery

Celery belongs to the parsley family, *Umbelliferae*, as do dill and other common spices and common allergens may be found.
Celery has been reported to cause multiple attacks of urticaria, angiooedema and also anaphylactic shock when eaten (8, 9).

The allergenic material on the discs consists of a mixture of fresh root and green leaf stalks from celery (*Apium*).

f86 Parsley

Parsley belongs to the *Umbelliferae* family together with celery, carrot (f31), coriander, dill, fennel and other common spices. Cross-reactivity within the family may be found. Parsley is a culinary herb often used as garnish. Allergic reactions such as anaphylactic shock are seen especially among atopic individuals allergic to weed pollens. The allergenic material on the discs consists of fresh parsley (*Petroselinum*).

Allergy to fruits is common with oranges (f33), tomatoes (f25), strawberries (f44) and melons seen as being the most common of such allergenic sources. The reactions are usually immediate appearing within minutes after ingestion of the fruit. Urticaria is probably the most common, but gastrointestinal symptoms and anaphylactic shock have been reported.

It has been observed clinically that the allergens are heat labile.

Allergic reactions to melons seem to occur among atopic individuals allergic to weed pollen, especially ragweed. As an explanation for the melon sensitivity-ragweed pollinosis syndrome, a strong cross-reactivity between ragweed and cantaloupe, suggesting common antigenic determinants, has been found (10).

The allergenic material on the discs consists of a mixture of honeydew (*Cucumis meloccharinus*) and cantaloupe (*C.melo cantalupensis*) melons.

Spices are well-known as being able to cause hypersensitivity reactions and to increase the symptoms in allergic patients. Recently it has been shown that they also may trigger IgE-mediated symptoms. In order to comprehend the incidence of hypersensitivity to food stuffs, a poll was taken of members of the Swedish National Association against Allergy. The results show that hypersensitivity to food stuffs, a poll was taken of members of the Swedish National Association against Allergy. The results show that hypersensitivity to spices is considered to be rather frequent as 30% of the patients reported spices to cause problems.

Table mustard is prepared from either seed of *Brassica nigra (Sinapis nigra)*, Brown, black or red mustard) or seeds of *Sinapis alba* (White mustard) or a mixture of both genera belonging to the *Cruciferae* (Mustard) family. Broccoli, Brussel sprouts, cabbage, cauliflower, horseradish, kohlrabi, radish, rutabaga and watercress belong to the same family. A possible cross-reactivity within this family cannot be excluded and an individual who reacts to mustard seed may also react to other *Cruciferae* members.

The ground seeds are also used in mayonnaise, different salad dressings, marinades, in some brands of ketchup, pickles, cumberland sauce etc. It is obvious that an allergy to mustard seed may be difficult to diagnose from the case history alone.
The allergenic material used to prepare the discs consists of a mixture of ground *Brassica* and *Sinapis* seeds.

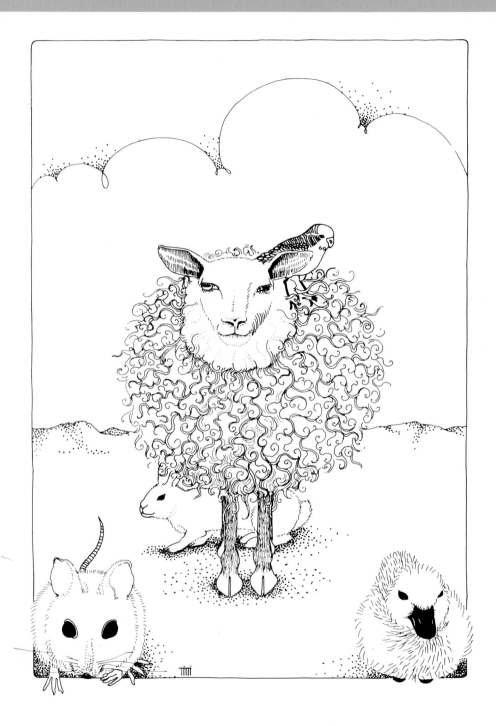

e71 Mouse epithelia

Hypersensitivity reactions to mouse epithelia are a common problem among laboratory workers and animal handlers. Allergy to mice has been reported in more than 10 % of laboratory workers, who may be unable to continue their work as a result. Identification of the relevant allergens and their source is necessary for control of this problem.

In certain areas mouse hair allergens present in house dust have been shown to be an important allergen in a high percentage of urban asthmatics (11).

The allergenic material on the discs consists of hair and skin-scrapings from CxBG-mice. Special care is taken to avoid contamination with serum and urine proteins.

e72 Mouse urine proteins

Laboratory workers and animal handlers not only may be sensitized to the epithelia but also to components in the mouse urine (12). The major allergen (MUP) is a prealbumin which causes allergy not only upon direct contact but also as a constituent in dust. Sensitization can follow inhalation of contaminated air-borne dust giving rise to specific IgE antibodies detectable by RAST (13). It was found that proper control of the collection and disposal of the animals' urine is necessary to minimize the likelihood of sensitization. The allergenic material on the discs consists of sterile urine from male CxBG-mice obtained by puncturing the bladder.

e76 Mouse serum proteins

It has clearly been demonstrated that there are at least two major allergens present in mouse skin, serum and urine (14). Individuals sensitive to mice may react predominately with either or all of these allergens. Urticarial reactions in and around a mouse bite have been reported. Furthermore, mild anaphylactic reactions involving hypotension, asthma and giant urticaria have been observed. Serum is regarded as a source of major allergens (14). Special precautions are taken to avoid contaminating the serum preparation with epithelia and urine proteins.

The allergenic material on the discs consists of unfractionated serum from Mouse Balb C.

e73 Rat epithelia

Laboratory workers and animal handlers often develop hypersensitivity to rat epithelia. Allergy to rats has been reported in more than 10 % of laboratory workers, the consequences of which may be that they are unable to continue their work (15). In fact, one may assume that up to 25 to 30 % of laboratory scientists and technicians who work closely with laboratory animals develop hypersensitivity to those animals.

The allergenic material on the discs consists of hair and skin-scrapings from Lou-rats.

e74 Rat urine proteins

The major allergen found in rat urine is an alpha-2-globulin. Positive skin prick and inhalation test reactions and RAST results for specific IgE antibodies have been obtained (12).

The allergenic material on the discs consists of sterile urine from Lou-rats obtained by puncturing the bladder.

e75 Rat serum proteins

It is speculated that the allergens found in serum are identical to those in the epithelia. However, it has been suggested that dander contains allergenic components that do not originate in serum (17).

The allergenic material on the discs consists of whole serum from Lou-rats.

e80 Goat epithelia

Extensive contact with goats may sensitize such people as veterinary surgeons, laboratory researchers, animal attendants and farmers.

Sheep and goat epithelia contain both common and unique allergens.

The allergenic material on the discs consists of hair and skin-scrapings. It contains trace amounts of serum proteins.

e81 Sheep epithelia

Frequent contact with sheep and sheep wool has been reported to sensitize highly predisposed individuals.

Wool is regarded as being a rather common allergen of importance not only for asthma and hay fever but also for eczema. Asthmatics who knit often suffer asthmatic attacks.

The allergenic material on the discs consists of hair and skin-scrapings. It contains trace amounts of serum proteins.

e82 Rabbit epithelia

Rabbits are extensively used as antisera-producing animals and people in close contact with these animals may become sensitized. There are good reasons to believe that rabbits from different species will show a high degree of cross-reactivity.

The allergenic material on the discs consists of hair and skin-scrapings. No rabbit gammaglobulin has been detected on the discs. False positive tests due to clinically irrelevant anti-gammaglobulin antibodies of the IgG type in the patient's serum might otherwise be seen (16).

e83 Swine epithelia

One factor that might cause allergic problems in people handling swine or swine products is swine epithelia. Allergy to swine epithelia has been described among farmers. The animals shed large amounts of dander.

The allergenic material on the discs consists of hair and skin-scrapings.

e84 Hamster epithelia

Asthma among animal handlers has often been traced back to hamsters whose allergens seem to be rather strong sensitizers. Due to the increasing popularity of these animals as pets, the allergic problems have now been transferred from animal handlers to pet-owners, particularly children.

The allergenic material on the discs consists of hair and skin-scrapings.

e70 Goose feathers

Down and feathers from geese and ducks are commonly used in bedding and warm sportswear.
The allergenic material on the discs consists of feathers and skin-scrapings from goose.

e85 Chicken feathers

Allergy to chicken feathers is seen not only after direct exposure to chickens but also after contact with pillows and mattresses containing such material. The allergenic material on the discs consists of feathers and down gathered from the nests of white leghorn.

e86 Duck feathers

The allergenic material on the discs consists of feathers and skin-scrapings from duck.

e87 Rat
e88 Mouse

"Total" ALLERGO-DISCS® have been produced where mouse epithelia, urine and serum proteins and rat epithelia, urine and serum proteins, respectively, have been coupled to discs for screening purposes. The same quality control criteria apply as for the single discs. Comparative studies show that few if any of the positive RAST tests to the corresponding epithelia-urine-serum proteins are missed by the "total" disc.

e78 Budgerigar feathers

The possibility of an allergic reaction to caged birds is easily overlooked, but these animals can cause serious problems. Allergic reactions, mainly symptoms from the respiratory tract, are seen in individuals keeping caged birds, either for pleasure or profit. Both immediate and delayed respiratory reactions have been reported.

The allergenic material on the discs consists of feathers and skin-scrapings from *Melopsittacus undulatus*, a small Australian budgerigar commonly kept as a pet (18).

e77 Budgerigar droppings

It has been shown that not only do the feathers and serum proteins contain antigens but also the droppings. There is a high level of cross-reactivity between allergens from budgerigar and other caged birds such as canary and finks.

The allergenic material on the discs consists of droppings from budgerigar. The material is sterilized by radiation before use.

e79 Budgerigar serum proteins

There is good evidence that budgerigar serum contains allergens that may sensitize predisposed individuals. The bird has glands that secrete a lipid-proteinaceous substance that the bird constantly applies to clean and weatherproof its feathers. This sebaceous material and saliva dry on the feathers and combine with powdery substances to create inhalant allergens.

The allergenic material on the discs consists of unfractionated serum from budgerigar (*Melopsittacus undulatus*).

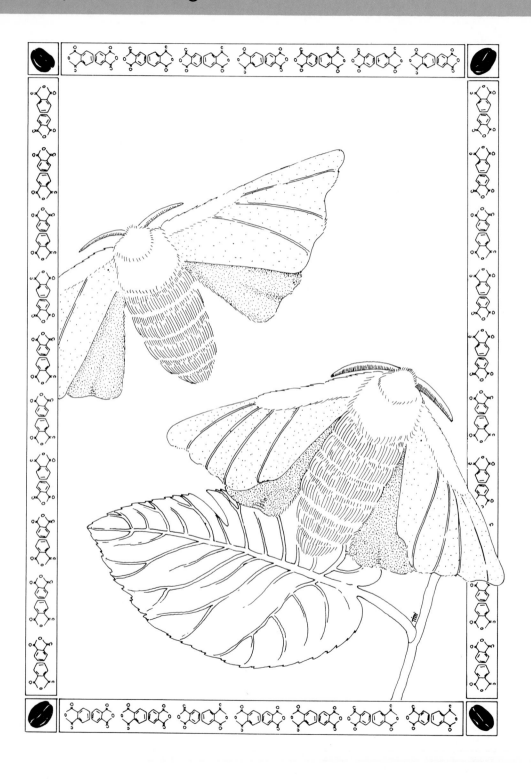

Studies from the coffee industry report that 10 % of workers exposed to the dust of the green coffee bean were found to have developed allergic symptoms, about half having asthma.

Green coffee from unroasted coffee beans produces a dust that contains highly immunogenic allergens. The true nature of the offending allergen or allergens remains to be elucidated. Green coffee beans from certain producers contain castor bean allergens as a contaminant which is another distinct group of very potent allergens (19). Workers in the coffee indsutry will, in high percentages, develop occupational allergies (hay fever and asthma) due to IgE-mediated allergy to this and other allergens (20). The allergens in green coffee dust are destroyed during the roasting process and cannot be detected in commercially available coffee products (21).

The allergenic material on the discs consists of selected preparations of green coffee bean dust. No contaminating castor bean allergens have been detected on the discs.

Castor bean allergen is regarded as one of the most potent allergens known and is capable of evoking severe allergic symptoms in sensitized individuals. As a result, allergy to castor bean has been found in a number of cases where the patients have been exposed to this agent.

Respiratory allergy to castor bean dust, first described among laboratory personnel and professional workers (farmers, dock workers, castor oil mill personnel), may develop in people who are not in direct contact with the beans. Employees in companies which import, prepare and distribute plant products and ingredients in health foods have shown positive RAST results to castor bean (22). The explanation could be that the sacks used for delivery of the products were contaminated with remnants from earlier contents of castor bean (19).

Epidemics of asthma have been described among citizens in areas where castor oil mills are in operation. Under appropriate conditions respiratory allergy to castor bean is apt to assume a recurrent character simulating pollinosis or mould allergy.

Clinically, symptoms are of the pollen allergy type such as rhinitis or asthma and in 25 % of the allergic cases, asthma is accompanied by urticaria. Castor bean allergic patients often present multiple sensitivities, allergy to house dust being the most frequently observed accompanying sensitization. Also cottonseed and flaxseed sensitivities have sometimes been observed.

Since castor is highly toxic, the use of provocation tests to confirm diagnosis is not feasible and skin tests can only be done at very low extract concentrations. Furthermore, castor bean meal contains ricin, a highly toxic protein that may induce pseudo-inflammatory delayed skin reaction; commercial extracts are not always free of this protein (22).

Thus where the clinical history raises the possibility of castor bean allergy, it is suggested that RAST using Castor bean ALLERGO-DISCS® is a suitable and reliable method to confirm the diagnosis.

The allergenic material on the discs consists of selected preparations of castor bean. No contaminating green coffee bean allergens have been detected on the discs.

Ispaghula has a high water-binding capacity and functions as a bulk laxative. The substance is stripped from the seeds of the Indian *Plantago* species. Ispaghula is an important occupational allergen giving rise to asthma and hay fever among exposed workers (23). The laxatives are commercially available under brand names such as Effersyl® (Stuart), Instant Mix Metamucil® (Searle), Konsyl® and L.A. Formula® (Burton, Parsons), Sof-Cil® (Zemmer), Syllamalt® (Abbott), Vi-Siblin® (Parke-Davis), and Lunelax® (Tika).

Hospital personnel exposed to the drug when administering to the patients inhale dust containing ispaghula and about 20 % develop asthma and hay fever (24). Sensitized individuals may react with asthma, rhinitis and gastrointestinal symptoms and even shock when taking the drugs orally.

There is little, if any, evidence that the drugs administered orally can sensitize. However, the most severe reactions have occurred in patients with respiratory symptoms when they have taken the drug orally for gastrointestinal malfunctions (25, 26). The allergen is resorbed intact from the gut and consequently every person taking the drug is at risk. This is probably especially true for children and young adults and those with an atopic constitution.

There are indications of allergenic cross-reactivity between the drug Ispaghula and pollens from other members of the *Plantago* family such as English plantain (*Plantago lanceolata*), and common plantain (*Plantago major*). It has been suggested that individuals allergic to English plantain should be carefully watched for manifestations of allergic symptomatology if they are using or in contact with *psyllium*-containing medications (27). The possible cross-reaction with pollens from *Plantago* should be stressed.

The allergenic material on the discs consists of a glycoprotein from the seeds of *Plantago ovata (psyllium)*.

k73 Silk waste

Cases of allergy to silk have been found among silk industry workers. Recently many patients in Europe have been reportedly sensitized upon contact with quilts stuffed with wild silk waste (28). Wild silk from silkworms of the species *Antheraea*, mostly living on oak leaves is used in heavy fabrics such as furniture coverings and draperies. The allergenic material on the discs consists of quilt stuffing containing silk waste supposedly from *Antheraea spp.*

k74 Silk

Textile products containing silk have been woven since the olden days but the literature contains few reports about allergic reactions to silk and silk products. When such cases have been reported the symptoms have been found in patients working in the silk industry (29). Silk fabrics are usually woven with silk from the cultivated silkworm *Bombyx mori* living on mulberry leaves. The allergenic material on the discs consists of cocoons from *Bombyx mori*.

In certain situations highly reactive, low molecular weight chemicals such as isocyanates and anhydrids can be allergenic. When the body is exposed to high concentrations, the chemicals can penetrate the mucosal membranes and after having bound to proteins act as haptens. Using human serum albumin (HSA) as the carrier it is possible to detect IgE-antibodies to these hapten-allergens.

Isocyanates

Isocyanates are widely used in the production of polyurethane plastics, glues and paints and hypersensitivity to these chemicals has been recognized for many years. Isocyanates are chemicals which are highly irritant to the respiratory passages and the eyes. A wide spectrum of respiratory illness has been described including both immediate and delayed reactions such as rhinitis, acute bronchitis, asthma, chronic bronchitis, bronchopneumonia and hypersensitivity pneumonitis. Up to 5 % of exposed workers have been reported to have developed asthma at work (30). After withdrawal from the contaminated environment recovery can be rapid and complete although there is now evidence that some of these patients have persistent asthma for years after removal from isocyanate exposure. Data concerning the potential hazards of isocyanates implicate both an immunological and a non-immunological mechanism behind the biological action. IgE antibodies specific to isocyanate haptens have been found in the sera of sensitized workers and 14 to 19 % of the cases can be classified as immunologically sensitized (31, 32). Symptom-free workers exposed to isocyanates in general have undetectable or low levels of IgE antibodies to the respective isocyanate.

RAST inhibition experiments indicate that antigenic determinants of the different isocyanate-HSA conjugates may be closely related structurally, but not identical (32). These findings of immunological cross-reactivity are supported by clinical hypersensitivity towards two or all three of the main industrial isocyanates, TDI, MDI and HDI. Routine serological screening of workers for tolyl-reactive antibodies may be of value in confirming suspected isocyanates exposure and in providing an early warning of developing hypersensitivity to isocyanates. Those at risk for isocyanate exposure include workers in polyurethane, foam, upholstery, spray painting, wire coating, metal rod coating, truck body insulation, plastic moulding, rubber workers, fabric coating, and persons applying artificial turf.

ALLERGO-DISCS® Isocyanate allergen products are available in a special kit containing one unit of 10 discs of the respective isocyanate hapten and one unit of 10 HSA discs.

The allergenic material on the discs consists of the respective isocyanate hapten conjugated to HSA. The conjugation has been prepared by reacting diisocyanate with HSA under mild conditions to avoid any formation of polymers. Each conjugate has been tested by several methods including direct RAST and RAST inhibition and has been found to be immunologically specific. For evaluation of the test results, HSA discs should be used to correct for any non-specific binding.

k75 TDI   Toluene diisocyanate

TDI is the most commonly used commercial isocyanate and widely used in the manufacture of polyurethane paints and plastics. The allergenic material on the disc consists of 2.4- and 2.6-toluene-diisocyanate hapten conjugated to HSA.

k76 MDI   Methylene diphenyl diisocyanate

Together with TDI and HDI, MDI is one of the most common isocyanates. The allergenic material on the disc consists of 4.4- diphenyl-methane-diisocyanate hapten conjugated with HSA.

k77 HDI   Hexamethylene diisocyanate

HDI together with TDI and MDI is one of the most common commercial isocyanates. The allergen on the discs is 1.6- hexa-methylene-diisocyanate hapten conjugated with HSA.

Ethylene oxide (EO) is commonly used for sterilization of heat-sensitive medical devices. EO-sterilized products may, however, contain EO residues and allergic reactions and anaphylaxis have been reported in patients receiving regular haemodialysis (35, 36).

EO is a highly reactive molecule and reacts with many compounds such as alcohols, organic acids, mercaptans and amines. It is therefore likely that EO may react *in vivo* with native proteins to create an immunogenic hapten. Thus, EO-specific IgE antibodies can be demonstrated in serum of EO-sensitive patients while sera from controls are negative in RAST (37, 38).

Patients exposed to tubings, syringes and other EO-sterilized devices may develop severe allergic reactions (rhinitis, breathlessness, chest oppression, urticaria) triggered by EO-specific IgE antibodies. ALLERGO-DISCS® Ethylene oxide makes it possible to detect such antibodies on a routine basis. The allergenic material on the discs consists of ethylene oxide conjugated to HSA. For evaluation of the test results HSA discs should be used to correct for any non-specific binding.

Ethylene oxide ALLERGO-DISCS® are available in a special kit containing one unit of 10 discs and one unit of 10 HSA discs.

* Synonyms: etenoxid, 1.2-epoxyethane, oxirane, dimethylene oxide

k79 Phthalic anhydride

Phthalic anhydride (PA) is an essential chemical in the manufacturing process of a variety of industrial products which include plasticizers, epoxy resins and paints and it has wide application in the chemical, plastic and electrical industries.

Bronchial obstructive disease from industrial chemicals accounts for a significant proportion of occupational respiratory disease. Only a few chemicals elicit symptoms that can be correlated with immunological reactivity. PA in high concentrations has probably a direct irritative affect on the bronchia. However, PA has also been shown to give rise to a high titre of specific IgE antibodies as measured by RAST (33). Furthermore, occasional occurrence of immediate-type reactions in patients undergoing haemodialysis therapy has been found and specific IgE antibodies to PA demonstrated. The reason for this sensitization seems to be that plastic materials in dialysis equipment leach PA which may provide the source of a hapten (34). The identification of specific IgE by RAST demonstrates that RAST can be a useful *in vitro* technique for identifying sensitization to this chemical.

The clinical findings reported are rhinorrhea, lacrimation, asthma and wheezing.

The allergenic material on the discs consists of phthalic anhydride conjugated to HSA. For evaluation of the test results HSA discs should be used to correct for any non-specific binding.

Phthalic anhydride ALLERGO-DISCS® are available in a special kit containing one unit of 10 discs and one unit of 10 HSA discs.

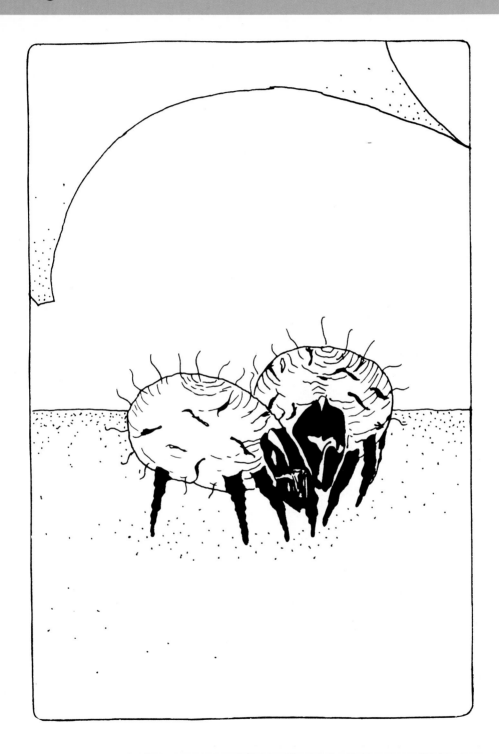

Acarus siro does not have any major allergens in common with
D. spp., (d1, d2) and thus no or very little cross-reactivity. Some cross-reactivity has been seen between *A. siro* and *Tyrophagus putrescentiae*.
A. siro feeds on *Alternaria, Streptomyces spp.* and *Penicillium*.

d71 *Lepidoglyphus destructor*

L. destructor does not have any major allergens in common with *D. spp.*
and no cross-reaction has been shown with *A. siro*. There does seem to be
cross-reactivity with *Glycyphagus domesticus,* d73. In a Canadian study,
L. destructor was the most common storage mite especially from spring to
fall (39). It feeds on *Alternaria* and *Penicillium*.

d72 *Tyrophagus putrescentiae*

As opposed to the other storage mites *Tyrophagus putrescentiae* shows
some cross-reactivity with *Dermatophagoides farinae* (40). Furthermore,
Tyrophagus putrescentiae shares some major allergens with *Acarus
siro* and consequently might show cross-reaction with that storage mite.
It is an important allergen source and should be considered when
Dermatophagoides pteronyssinus is thought to be a problem.

d73 *Glycyphagus domesticus*

This mite of the *Glycyphagidae* family is found in foods, grains, in
warehouses and other storage areas. In homes it thrives in infested food
stuffs and in damp areas where it feeds on moulds. The allergen discs may
contain some traces of yeast proteins from the growth media.

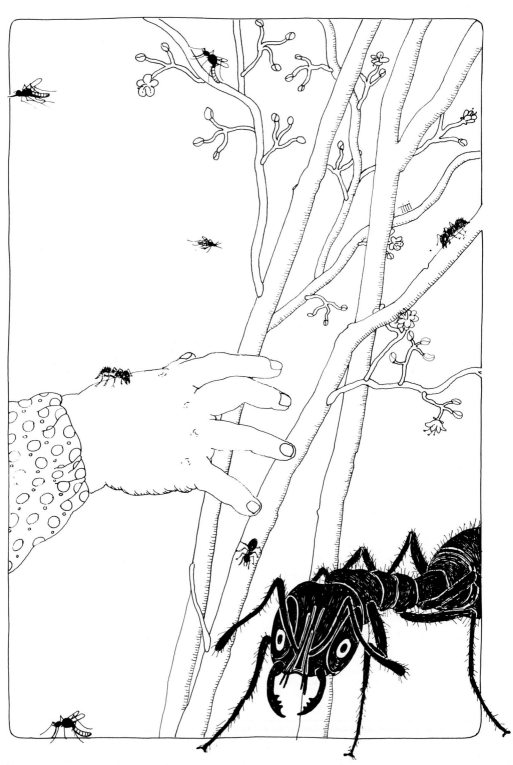

The fire ant is a stinging and biting ant common in South America and the southern United States. The insect attacks by biting to secure itself, then inserts its stinging apparatus which contains the venom. The sting gives a burning sensation followed by a local pustular type of reaction. Systemic reactions after a sting have been reported (41). The venom contains several alkaloids with potent biological properties but very little, less than 1 %, or no protein. There seems to be considerable allergenic similarities among ants of the genus *Solenopsis* but the venom of the fire ant differs from that of *Hymenoptera* insects.

There is a cross-reaction with insects of the order *Hymenoptera*. About 14 % of European patients allergic to Yellow jacket, *Vespula spp.*, are RAST-positive to Fire ant, a figure which increases to 27 % after venom immunotherapy (42). Honey bee (*Apis mellifera*) patients do not seem to show this cross-reaction. See also Phadebas RAST®/Phadezym RAST® venom allergen discs i1-i5.

The allergenic material on the discs consists of whole bodies of Fire ant, *Solenopsis invicta*. In the US it is called Imported fire ant.

i71 *Aedes communis*
Common mosquito

The family *Culicidae* (stinging mosquitoes) to which *Aedes communis* belongs, is found almost all over Europe, in North America, Asia and Japan.

Respiratory allergy to *Aedes* fragments in dust has been reported, but hypersensitivity to stings cannot be excluded. Large local reactions as a result of a sting are, in the majority of cases, triggered by non-allergic mechanisms. Mechanisms involved in sting reactions are under investigation.

The cross-reactivity within the *Culicidae* family is most probably extensive, and a certain degree of cross-reactivity with other families cannot be excluded.

The allergenic material on the discs consists of whole insects of *Aedes communis*.

i72 *Cladotanytarsus Lewisi*
Green nimitti

Cladotanytarsus Lewisi (Green nimitti, Sudan fly) belongs to the *Chironomidae* family which is distributed world-wide. The allergenic respiratory problems associated with *C. Lewisi* have mainly been reported in people living close to the Nile in northern and central Sudan and around Lake Victoria in Uganda. In these areas peak emergencies which reach plague proportions in some years usually seem to occur in the period of low discharge of the Nile, in the months following the late summer/autumn rains. The symptoms reported are mainly bronchial asthma and rhinitis.

The allergens have been extensively investigated. The results indicate that the major allergen is likely to be chironomid haemoglobin. A considerable degree of cross-reactivity has been found between *C. Lewisi* and *Chironomus Thummi Th*. This strongly indicates that similar antigenic determinants are probably present in both species. If this finding is substantiated, chironomids, because of their world-wide distribution, may be recognized as an important cause of environmental and occupational allergy.

The allergenic material on the discs consists of whole insects of *Cladotanytarsus Lewisi*.

The genus *Chironomus* is represented by a great number of species in fresh water habitats all over the world. Recently it was deduced that *C. Thummi Th.* and *C. riparius* are synonymous. The most correct name today would be *C. riparius.*

It is found all over Europe and this species is with high certainty also found in North America. The reason for this dubious statement is that the characterization and identification is extremely difficult.

The allergenic problems, however, are mainly due to the fact that larvae of this species are extensively used as fish bait for aquarium fishes. The allergens have a high tendency to sensitize. Several cases of severe respiratory and rhinoconjunctival symptoms have been reported, some of which are of special interest as no previous exposure to larvae of the Blood worm had been established. However, some of the patients reported symptoms while in an agricultural environment. Studies are ongoing to investigate possbile cross-reactivity with allergens found in a farming milieu.

Furthermore, it has been observed that patients, when skin tested, have positive reactions only to Blood worm larvae and shrimp. It could be possible that a certain cross-reactivity exists between these larvae and crustaceans or that some individuals develop allergy against certain arthropodes.

The allergenic material on the discs consists of freeze-dried larvae of *Chironomus Thummi Th.*

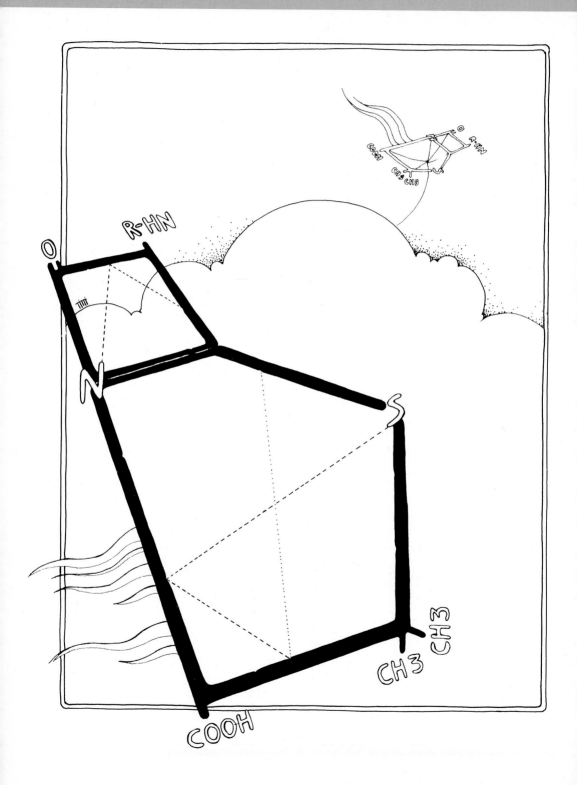

c70 Insulin, porcine

The allergenic material on the discs consists of monocomponent insulin from swine.

c71 Insulin, bovine

The allergenic material on the discs consist of insulin of bovine origin purified by chromatography to "single peak" quality.

c73 Insulin, human

The recently introduced recombinant DNA-technique for insulin production has made it possible to produce human insulin. Even if the porcine and bovine insulin structure only shows minor differences in the amino acid sequence as compared to human insulin, it has been aimed at producing human insulin mainly for two reasons: It may be difficult to cover the future requirement for all diabetics with the animal products; and, the immunogenicity is hoped to be less with the recombinant human insulin, thereby resulting in less allergic reactions. The hope of eliminating allergic reactions has unfortunately come to nought and it has been demonstrated that specific IgE antibodies can be produced to allergens unique to the insulin molecule as shown in a patient who developed a generalized reaction to human insulin (43).

The allergenic material on the discs consists of human insulin, Humulin® Regular 40 IU/ml, an original product from Eli Lilly, USA and sold under license by KabiVitrum, Sweden.

The literature contains a number of case reports of human seminal fluid allergy. There are indications of the presence of sensitizing components which may be common to all semen but the structure of the allergenic components has not yet been determined. In several cases IgE antibody has been shown to be responsible for mediating the allergic reactions. Several articles have described patients with various allergic responses, ranging from local pruritus to systemic anaphylaxis (43).

Due to the lack of appropriate testing reagents and the sensitive nature of the issue there are good reasons to believe that the prevalence of this problem is underestimated.

The allergenic material on the discs consists of semen specimens obtained from healthy, fertile donors. The samples are centrifuged to remove spermatozoa. The seminal plasma specimens are then pooled and gelfiltrated on Sephacryl® S-200 (Pharmacia Biotechnology, Uppsala, Sweden) before coupling to the discs.

1. Villaveces J.W.
Tree allergy and the street-tree guide.
J Asthma Res 22 (1973) p. 42.

2. Singh A.B. and Babu C.R.
Studies on pollen allergy in Delhi.
Diurnal periodicity of common
allergenic pollen.
Allergy 35 (1980) p. 311.

3. Targow A.M.
The mulberry tree: A neglected factor
in respiratory allergy in southern
California.
Ann Allergy 29 (1971) p. 318.

4. Langeland T.
A clinical and immunological study of
allergy to hen's egg white.
Allergy 38 (1983) p. 399.

5. Heiner D.C., Goldstein G. and Rose B.
Immunochemical studies of selected
subjects with wheat intolerance.
J Allergy 45 (1970) p. 333.

6. Baldo B.A. and Wrigley C.W.
IgE antibodies to wheat flour
components. Clin Allergy 8 (1978)
p. 109.

7. Fine A.J.
Hypersensitivity reaction to kiwi fruit
(Chinese gooseberry, Actinidia
chinensis). J Allergy Clin Immunol 68
(1981) p. 235.

8. Kauppinen K., Kousa M. and
Reunala T.
Aromatic plants - A cause of severe
attacks of angiooedema and urticaria.
Contact Dermat 6 (1980) p. 251.

9. Forsbeck M. and Ros A.-M.
Anaphylactoid reactions to celery.
Contact Dermat 5 (1979) p. 191.

10. Anderson L.B., Dreyfuss E.M., Logan
J., Johnstone D.E. and Glaser J.
Melon and banana sensitivity coincident
with ragweed pollinosis.
J Allergy 45 (1970) p. 310.

11. Lim D.T. and Ganju A.
Reaginic sensitivity to Mus musculus
extract in a group of Chicago urban
asthmatics.
Ann Allergy 44 (1980) p. 267.

12. Taylor A.N., Longbottom J.L. and
Pepys J.
Respiratory allergy to urine proteins of
rats and mice. Lancet ii (1977) p. 847.

13. Edwards E.G., Lee D., Beeson M.F.,
Dewdney J. M. and Spackman D.A.
Development and validation of RAST for
the detection of specific human IgE
antibody directed against laboratory
animal urinary proteins.
Int Arch Allergy appl Immunol 71 (1983)
p. 53.

14. Siraganian R.P. and Sandberg A.L.
Characterization of mouse allergens.
J Allergy Clin Immunol 63 (1979)
p. 435.

15. Lincoln T.A., Bolton N.E. and
Garrett A.S.Jr.
Occupational allergy to animal dander
and sera. J Occ Med 16 (1974) p. 465.

16. Foucard T., Bennich H., Johansson
S.G.O. and Lundkvist U.
Human antibodies to bovine
globulin. Occurrence in immunological
disorders and influence on allergy radio-
immunoassays.
Int Arch Allergy appl Immunol 48 (1975)
p. 812.

17. Ohman J.L., Lowell F.C. and Bioch K.J.
Allergens of mammalian origin. J Allergy
Clin Immunol 55 (1975) p. 16.

18. *Faux J.S., Wide L., Hargreave F .E., Longbottom J.L. and Pepys J.* Immunological aspects of respiratory allergy in budgerigar *(Melopsittacus undulatus)* fanciers. Clin Allergy 1 (1971) p. 149.

19. *Karr R.M., Lehrer S.B., Butcher B.T. and Salvaggio J.E.* Coffee worker's asthma: A clinical appraisal using the radioallergosorbent test. J Allergy Clin Immunol 62 (1978) p. 143.

20. *Bernton H.S.* On occupational sensitization. A hazard to the coffee industry. JAMA 223 (1973) p. 1146.

21. *Layton L.L., Greene F.C., Panzani R. and Corse J.W.* Allergy to green coffee. Failure of patients allergic to green coffee to react to chlorogenic acid, roasted coffee, or orange. J Allergy 36 (1965) p. 84.

22. *Göthe C.-J., Wieslander G., Ancker K. and Forsbeck M.* Buckwheat allergy: Health food, an inhalation health risk. Allergy 38 (1983) p. 155.

23. *Busse W.D. and Schreutwetter W.F.* Asthma from *psyllium* in laxative manufacture. Ann Intern Med 83 (1975) p. 361.

24. *Machado L., Zetterström O. and Fagerberg E.* Occupational allergy in nurses to a bulk laxative. Allergy 34 (1979) p. 51.

25. *Suhonen R., Kantola I. and Björkstén F.* Anaphylactic shock due to ingestion of *psyllium* laxative. Allergy 38 (1983) p. 363.

26. *Machado L. and Ståhlenheim G.* Respiratory symptoms in ispaghula-allergic nurses after oral challenge with ispaghula suspension. Allergy 39 (1984) p. 65.

27. *Rosenberg S., Landay R., Klotz S.D. and Fireman P.* Serum IgE antibodies to *psyllium* in individuals allergic to *psyllium* and English plantain. Ann Allergy 48 (1982) p. 294.

28. *Häcki M., Wüthrich B. and Hauser M.* Wildseide: ein aggressives Inhalationsallergen (Wild silk: a strong inhalation allergen, English summary). Dtsch med Wschr 107 (1982) p. 166.

29. *Kobayashi S.* Occupational asthma due to inhalation of pharmacological dusts and other chemical agents with some reference to other occupational asthmas in Japan. In Allergology Proc. VIII Int. Congr. Allergol. eds. Y. Yamamura et al. Excerpta Medica, Amsterdam, 1973 p. 127.

30. *Butcher B.T., Karr R.M., O'Neil C.E., Wilson M.R.,* Pharmarajan V., Salvaggio J.E. and Weill H. Inhalation challenge and pharmacologic studies of toluene di-isosyanate (TDI)-sensitive workers. Allergy Clin Immunol 64 (1979) p. 146.

31. Butcher B.T., O'Neil C.E., Reed M.A.
     and Salvaggio J.E.
     Radio-allergo-sorbent testing of toluene
     di-isocyanate-reactive individuals using
     p-tolyle isocyanate antigen.
     J Allergy Clin Immunol 66 (1980) p. 213.

32. Baur X.
     Immunologic cross-reactivity between
     different albumin-bound isocyanates.
     J Allergy Clin Immunol 71 (1983) p. 197.

33. Maccia C.A., Bernstein I.L., Emmett
     E.A. and Brooks S.M.
     In vitro demonstration of specific IgE in
     phthalic anhydride hypersensitivity.
     Am Rev Resp Dis 113 (1976) p. 701.

34. Patterson R., Zeiss C.R., Roxe D.,
     Pruzansky J.J., Roberts M. and Harris
     K.E.
     Antibodies in hemodialysis patients
     against hapten-protein and hapten-
     erythrocytes.
     J Lab Clin Med 96 (1980) p. 347.

35. Nicholls A.J. and Platts-Mills T.A.E.
     Anaphylactoid reactions due to
     haemodialysis, haemofiltration, or
     membrane plasma separation.
     BMJ 285 (1982) p. 1607.

36. Poothullil J., Shimizu A., Day R.P. and
     Dolovich J.
     Anaphylaxis from the product(s) of
     ethylene oxide gas. Ann Intern Med 82
     (1975) p. 58.

37. Dolovich J. and Bell B.
     Allergy to a product(s) of ethylene oxide
     gas. Demonstration of IgE and IgG
     antibodies and hapten specificity.
     J Allergy Clin Immunol 62 (1978) p. 30.

38. Belin L., Wass U. and Delin K.
     Hapten sensitization to ethylene oxide.
     J Allergy Clin Immunol 73 (1984) p. 164.

39. Warren C.P.W., Holford-Strevens V.
     and Sinha R.N.
     Sensitization in a grain handler to the
     storage mite Lepidoglyphus destructor.
     Ann Allergy 50 (1983) p. 30.

40. Green W.F. and Woolcock A.J.
     Tyrophagus putrescentiae:
     An allergenically important mite.
     Clin Allergy 18 (1978) p. 135.

41. Lockey R.F.
     Systemic reactions to stinging ants.
     J Allergy Clin Immunol 54 (1974) p. 132

42. Johansson S.G.O. and Lockey R.F.
     RAST studies of allergy to imported fire
     ant (IFA) (Solenopsis invicta).
     J Allergy Clin Immunol 71 (1983) p. 138.

43   Child F. and Johansson S.G.O.
     IgE antibody studies in a case of
     generalized allergic reaction to human
     insulin.
     Allergy 39 (1984) p. 3601.

1–17 References

1. Arbesman C.E., Reisman R.E. and Wypych J.I.
Allergenic potency of bee antigens measured by RAST inhibition. Clin Allergy 6 (1976) p. 587-594.

2. Swoboda B., Grond K. and Ludvan M.
IgE-Bestimmungen (RIST, RAST) und hauttest bei Pollinosis-Patienten. Z Hautkr 50 (1975) p. 441-447.

3. Gleich G.J., Leiferman K.M and Jones R.T.
Use of the radioallergosorbent test for the determination of the potency and cross-reactivity of allergy extracts. In: Advances in diagnosis of allergy: RAST Proc 1st N. Amer. Conf on RAST Palm Springs, Calif. 1975. Ed by R Evans III. Miami, Fla. (Symposia specialists) 1975 p. 57-83.

4. Schneeberger H.W., Seibert E., Steinhausen D. and Forck G.
Die Bedeutung des Radioallergo-sorbenstestes (RAST) im Vergleich mit dem Intrakutantest bei der Diagnose allergischer Erkrankungen. Acta Allergol 30 (1975) p. 411-422.

5. Bernstein I.L., Perera M., Gallagher J., Michael J.G. and Johansson S.G.O.
In vitro cross-allergenicity of major aeroallergenic pollens by the radioallergosorbent technique. J Allergy Clin Immunol 57 (1976) p. 141-152.

6. Leiferman K.M. and Gleich G.J.
The cross-reactivity of IgE antibodies with pollen allergens. I. Analyses of various species of grass pollens. J Allergy Clin Immunol 58 (1976) p. 129-139.

7. Shinomiya K., Mikawa H., Hirao T. and Yoshida T.
Atopic antibodies in sera of children. Part IV. Clinical application of radioallergosorbent test (RAST) for diagnosis of allergic children in Japan. Ann Paediatr Jpn 22 (1976) p. 12-23.

8. Miller A.C.M.L.
A comparative trial of hyposensitization in 1973 in the treatment of hay fever using Pollinex and Alava-P. Clin Allergy 6 (1976) p. 551-556.

9. Miller A.C.M.L.
A trial of hyposensitization in 1974/5 in the treatment of hay fever using glutaraldehyde-pollen-tyrosine adsorbate. Clin Allergy 6 (1976) p. 557-561.

10. Endres P.
Screening von Asthmatikern mittels IgE-Bestimmung und Erfassung eines Spektrums allergospezifischer IgE-Antikörper. Med Welt 28 (1977) p. 1797-1800.

11. Wortman F.
Oral hyposensitization of children with pollinosis or house-dust asthma. Allergol Immunopathol 5 (1977) p. 15-26.

12. Palmer W.R. and Balacescu A.
A multi-centre trial of pollen-tyrosine adsorbate. Acta Allergol 32 (1977) p. 44-57.

13. Düngemann H.
Karenz – Expositionsprophylaxe. Atemweg Lungenk 4 (1978) p. 7-14.

14. Kersten W. and Hoek G.T.
Der wert des Radio-Allergo-Sorbent-Tests (RAST) bei der Diagnose der Pollinose. Fortschr Med 96 (1978) p. 597-599.

15. Kalveram K.J. and Forck G.
Untersuchungen zum rationelleren Einsatz des Radio-Allergo-Sorbent-Test (RAST). Allergologie 2 (1979) p. 90-93.

16. Pullman H., Hasse A., Bloedhorn H., Gottmann-Lückerath I., Florescu S. and Schlaeger M.
RAST bei Gräser-Pollen-Allergikern zur Frage des repräsentativen Grases. Z Hautkr 54 (1979) p. 232-236.

17. Oprée W.
Die spezifität der IgE-antikörper als immunologisches Reifungsproblem. Z Hautkr 54 (1979) p. 225-231.

18. Becker S., Neumann M. and Veltman G.
Kutane oder intrakutane Testung in der diagnostik der Inhalationsallergien? Vergleichende Untersuchung Pollenfreier und Pollenhaltiger Allergenextrakte in der Kutanen und Intrakutanen Testung. II. Untersuchung der Pollenhaltigen Allergenextrakte. Med Welt 31 (1980) p. 868-873.

19. Ballow M. and Mendelson L.
Specific immunoglobulin E antibodies in tear secretions of patients with vernal conjuntivitis. J Allergy Clin Immunol 66 (1980) p. 112-118.

20. Løwenstein H.
Cross reactions among pollen antigens. Allergy 35 (1980) p. 198-200.

21. Brown W.G., Halonen M.J., Kaltenborn W.T. and Barbee R.A.
The relationship of respiratory allergy, skin test reactivity and serum IgE in a community population sample. J Allergy Clin Immunol 63 (1979) p. 328-335.

22. Hobday J.D.
The incidence of pollen sensitivities on skin test and bronchial challenge in asthmatic children in Perth, Western Australia. Med J Aust 1 (1972) p. 161-164.

23. Virchow C., Roth A. and Möller E.
IgE antibodies to house dust, mite, animal allergens and moulds in house dust hypersensitivity. Clin Allergy 6 (1979) p. 147-154.

24. Data on file G49. Monitoring specific IgE antibody levels in patients with hypersensitivity to cockroach antigens.

25. Lee T.H., Kay A.B., Douglas A.C. and Kemeny M.
The treatment of Hymenoptera sensitivity with whole body extract: A false sense of security. Lancet (1981:2) p. 301.

26. Pidock N.B., El-Aaser A., El-Sabei I. and Cooper E.H.
Immunoglobulin A and G levels and IgE responses to Schistosomiasis and Ascaris in Egyptians with bladder cancer. Draft, in press (1983).

27. Church J.A., Kleban D.G. and Bellanti J.A.
Serum immunoglobulin E concentrations and radioallergosorbent test in children with atopic dermatitis. Pediatr Res 10 (1976) p. 97-99.

28. Merrett T.G., Merrett J. and Cookson J.B.
Allergy and parasites: The measurement of total and specific IgE levels in urban and rural communities in Rhodesia. Clin Allergy 6 (1976) p. 131-134.

29. Cukor P., Woehler M.E., Persiani C. and Fermin A.
Iodinated versus fluorescent labelling in the radioallergosorbent test (RAST) for the determination of serum IgE levels. J Immunol Meth 12 (1976) p. 183-192.

30. Sobotka A.K., Franklin R.M., Adkinson N.F. Jr., Valentine M., Baer H. and Lichtenstein L.
Allergy to insect stings. II. Phospholipase A: The major allergen in honeybee venom. J Allergy Clin Immunol 57 (1976) p. 29-40.

31. Nagaya H., Lee S.K., R eddy P.M., Pascual H., Jerome D., Sadai J., Gupta S. and Lauridsen J.
Lymphocyte response to grass pollen antigens: A correlation with radioallergosorbent test and effect of immunotherapy. Ann Allergy 39 (1977) p. 246-252.

32. Hoffman D.R., Shipman W.H. and Babin D.
Allergens in bee venom. II. Two new high molecular weight allergenic specificities. J Allergy Clin Immunol 59 (1977) p. 147-153.

33. Pascual H.C., Reddy P.M., Nagaya H., Lee S.L., Lauridsen J. and Gupta S. Agreement between radioallergo-sorbent test and skin test. Ann Allergy 39 (1977) p. 325-327.

34. Data on file G 55. Performance of discs on sera from food-allergic patients from USA.

35. Paull B.R., Yunginger J.W. and Gleich G.J. Melittin: An allergen of honeybee venom. J Allergy Clin Immunol 59 (1977) p. 334-338.

36. Adalioglu G.A., Özkaragoez K. and Saraçlar Y. Comparison between rat mast cell degranulation test and allergic skin tests in children with atopic diseases. Turk J Pediatr 20 (1978) p. 1-2.

37. Zeiss C.R., Levitz D. and Suszko I. Quantitation of IgE antibody specific for ragweed and grass allergens: Binding of radiolabelled allergens by solid-phase bound IgE. J Allergy Clin Immunol 62 (1978) p. 83-90.

38. Hoffman D.R. Allergens in bee venom. III. Identification of allergen B of bee venom as an acid phosphatase. J Allergy Clin Immunol 59 (1977) p. 364-366.

39. Rappaport I., dePonce D., Sogn D. and Wang Y.Y. On the correlation between RAST and the allergy intradermal test. Ann Allergy 43 (1979) p. 1-7.

40. Nagaya H. Relationship between antigen-specific IgE antibody (RAST) and total serum IgE levels. Ann Allergy 43 (1979) p. 267-270.

41. Knight A., Underdown B.J., Connell J.T., Nedzelski J. and Elie R. Immunological parameters in perennial rhinitis. Clin Allergy 9 (1979) p. 159-166.

42. Hamburger R.N. Allergies in infants — perhaps they can be prevented. Consultant 9 (1979) p. 23-25, 29.

43. Pauli G., Bessot J.C., Kjelladi A. and Thierry R. Apport du RAST direct et de l'inhibition du RAST a l'identification des allèrgenes de la poussière. Rev Fr Allergol 20 (1980) p. 23-28.

44. Kniker W.T. Essai de standardisation des tests cutanés. Etudes corrélative entre le test par multipuncture, la détermination du seuil de réaction intradermique et le RAST avec les pneumallergènes. Rev Fr Allergol 20 (1980) p. 177-184.

45. Hamburger R.N. Development of atopic allergy in children. Int Allergy Symp., Uppsala, Sept 24-26, 1980 p. 30-34.

46. Nelson H. S. The selection of atopic allergens. J Asthma Res 18 (1981) p. 23-26.

47. Stempel D.A., Davis V.L., Morissey L.J. and Helms R.W. Seasonal variations of serum IgE levels in normal children. Ann Allergy 47 (1981) p. 14-16.

48. Barbee R.A., Brown W.G., Kaltenborn W. and Halonen M. Allergen skin-test reactivity in a community population sample: Correlation with age, histamine skin reactions, and toal serum immunoglobulin E. J Allergy Clin Immunol 68 (1981) p. 15-19.

49. Barbee R.A., Halonen M., Lebowitz M. and Burrows B. Distribution of IgE in a community population sample: Correlations with age, sex, and allergen skin test reactivity. J Allergy Clin Immunol 68 (1981) p. 106-111.

50. *Subirá M.L. and Oehling A.*
Diagnostic value of total IgE and antigen specific IgE using RAST in pollinosis. Allergol Immunopathol 3 (1975) p. 9-16.

51. *Pepys J., Roth A. and Carroll K.B.*
RAST, skin and nasal tests and the history in grass pollen allergy. Clin Allergy 5 (1975) p. 431-442.

52. *Aukrust L., Einarsson R., Öhman S. and Johansson S.G.O.*
Crossed radioimmunoelectrophoretic studies of bee venom allergens. Allergy 37 (1982) p. 265-271.

53. Data on file G 55. Collaborative study of antigens for immunodiagnosis of Schistosomiasis. Pharmacia, WHO, 1981.

54. *Morr H., Tachezy H. and von Wichert P.*
Allergenspezifisches IgE und Asthma bronchiale. Pneumonologie 152 (1975) p. 57-64.

55. *Halpern G.M., Lévy C., Garcelon M. and Dabouraud D.*
Approche diagnostique actuelle an allergologie respiratoire. Med Hyg 33 (1975) p. 41-45.

56. *Wagatsuma Y., Yakura H., Nakayama E., Wakisaka A., Aizawa M., Miyata M., Matsuyama R., Sato M. and Itakura K.*
Inheritance of asthma in families and its linkage to HLA haplotypes. Acta Allergol 31 (1976) p. 455-462.

57. *Blands J., Diamant B., Kallos P., Kallos-Deffner L. and Løwenstein H.*
Flour allergy in bakers. I. Identification of allergenic fractions in flour and comparison of diagnostic methods. Int Arch Allergy appl Immunol 52 (1976) p. 392-406.

58. *Hoffman D.R.*
Allergens in *Hymenoptera* venom. V. Identification of some of the enzymes and demonstration of multiple allergens in yellow jacket venom. Ann Allergy 40 (1978) p. 171-176.

59. *Werett D.J. and King L.A.*
Allergy profiles from bloodstains. Clin Allergy 6 (1976) p. 75-77.

60. *Houba, Václav*
Immunological investigation of tropical parasitic diseases. Churchill Livingston, Edinburgh London New York, 1980.

61. *Jarisch R.*
Rhinitis Allergica - verbessert der Radioallergosorbenttest die Diagnostik. Wien Klin Wochenschr 90 (1978) p. 313-316.

62. *King T.P., Sobotka A.K., Alagon A., Kochoumian L. and Lichtenstein L.M.*
Protein allergens of white-faced hornet, yellow hornet, and yellow jacket venoms. Biochemistry 17 (1978) p. 5165-5174.

63. *Malmberg H. and Holopainen E.*
Nasal smear as a screening test for immediate-type nasal allergy. Allergy 34 (1979) p. 331-337.

64. *Goto A.*
Half volume measurement of special IgE antibody. Radioisotopes 28 (1979) p. 766-768 (In Japan).

65. *Frostad A.B., Grimmer O., Sandvik L. and Aas K. Hyposensitization.*
Comparing a purified (refined) allergen preparation and a crude aqueous extract. Allergy 35 (1980) p. 81-95.

66. *Michel F.B., Bousquet J., Greillier P., Robinet-Levy M. and Coulomb Y.*
Comparison of cord blood immunoglobulin E concentrations and maternal allergy for the prediction of atopic diseases in infancy. J Allergy Clin Immunol 65 (1980) p. 422-430.

67. *Shepherd G.W., Elliott W.B. and Arbesman C.E.*
Fractionation of bee venom. I. Preparation and characterization of four antigenic components. Prep Biochem 4 (1974) p. 71-88.

68–83 References

68. Nelson H.S.
Long-term immunotherapy with aqueous and aluminum-precipitated grass extracts. Ann Allergy 45 (1980) p. 333-347.

69. de Filippi I., Yman L. and Schröder H.
Clinical accuracy of updated version of the Phadebas RAST® test. Ann Allergy 46 (1981) p. 249-255.

70. Santrach P.J., Parker J.L., Jones R.T. and Yuninger J.W.
Diagnostic and therapeutic applications of a modified radioallergosorbent test and comparison with the conventional radioallergosorbent test. J Allergy Clin Immunol 67 (1981) p. 97-104.

71. Noster U.
Die Bedeutung des Radioallergosorbenttests (RAST) in der Praxis der Allergiediagnostik. Therapiewoche 27 (1977) p. 4403-4410.

72. Yman L.
Botanical relations and immunological cross-reactions in pollen allergy. 2nd edition. Revised and enlarged. 1982. Pharmacia Diagnostics AB, Uppsala, Sweden.

73. Hoffman D.R. and McDonald C.A.
Allergens in Hymenoptera venom. VII. Species specific reactivity to yellow jacket venoms. Ann Allergy 47 (1981) p. 23-27.

74. Gleich G.J., Campbell A.R., Gleich M.C. and Swedlund H.A.
Differences in the reactivity of short and giant ragweed with immunoglobulin E antibodies. J Allergy Clin Immunol 65 (1980) p. 110-117.

75. Shephard E.G., MacFarlane C.M. and Joubert J.R.
A radioallergosorbent test (RAST) for Ascaris lumbricoides. Allergy 37 (1982) p. 231-239.

76. Tovey E.R., Chapman M.D. and Platts-Mills T.A.E.
Mite faeces are a major source of house dust allergens. Nature 289 (1981) p. 592-593.

77. Göthe C-J., Wieslander G., Ancker K. and Forsbeck M.
Buckwheat allergy: Health food, an inhalation health risk. Allergy 38 (1983) p. 155-159.

78. Hoffman D.R. and McDonald C.A.
Allergens in Hymenoptera venom. VIII. Immunologic comparison of venoms from six species of Vespula (Yellow jackets). Ann Allergy 48 (1982) p. 78-81.

79. Ben Ismael., Mogahed A., Boiteau A., Sainte-Laudy J., Carme B., Danis M. and Gentilini M.
Evaluation des immunoglobulines E dans l'hydatidase. Méd Mal Infect 12 (1982) p. 292-296.

80. Data on file G46. A new modified RAST® system. Comparison of previous and new Phadebas RAST system and the significance of the new in vitro test system compared to clinical history and in vivo test procedures. Contributors from Sweden, Norway, Switzerland, Finland, England, West Germany, France Denmark. 1979.

81. Hoffman D.R.
The specificities of human IgE antibodies combining with cereal grains. Immunochem 12 (1975) p. 535-538.

82. Blanchard G.C. and Gardner R.
The characterization of some of the antigens and allergens in ragweed pollen. Ann Allergy 39 (1977) p. 253-262.

83. Radermecker M., Bekhti A., Poncelet E. and Salmon J.
Serum IgE levels in protozoal and helminthic infections. Int Arch Allergy 47 (1974) p. 285-295.

84. Turner K.J., Stewart G.A., Sharp A.H. and Czarny D.
Standardization of allergen extracts by inhibition of RAST, skin test and chemical composition. Clin Allergy 10 (1980) p. 441-450.

85. Bryant D.H., Burns M.W. and Lazarus L.
The correlation between skin test, bronchial provocation tests and the serum level of IgE specific for common allergens in patients with asthma. Clin Allergy 5 (1975) p. 145-157.

86. Kleinhans D.
Bienentoxin-allergie-radio-allergo-sorbens-test (RAST) und Hauttest-ergebnisse. Dermatologie 6 (1977) p. Spalt 1-9.

87. Data on file G55. Research report. Phadebas RAST® compared with in vivo tests in the diagnosis of weed and tree pollen-hypersensitivity. Switzerland.

88. Müller U., Spiess J., Patrizzi R., Roth A. and Hoigne R.
Die bedeutung serologischer untersuchungen für diagnose und therapie der Insektenstickallergie. Schweiz Med Wochenschr 107 (1977) p. 1747-1749.

89. Basomba A., Juneskans B., Dahlström B., Einarsson R., Nilsson G., and Dreborg S.
Biological standardization (BS) of allergen extracts. XII Congress of the European Academy of Allergology and Clinical Immunology, Rome, Sept. 25-30, 1983.

90. Müller U., Spiess J. and Roth A.
Serological investigations in Hymenoptera sting allergy: IgE and haemagglutinating antibodies against bee venom in patients with bee sting allergy, bee keepers and non-allergic blood donors. Clin Allergy 7 (1977) p. 147-154.

91. Chodirker W.B. and Piotrowska A.
Allergy testing: Comparison of skin and in vitro tests of allergic reagin. CMAJ 116 (1977) p. 1254-1257.

92. Müller U., Roth A., Yman L. and Patrizzi R.
Use of RAST technique in wasp sting hypersensitivity. Cross-reactions between various insect antigens are specially considered. Allergy 33 (1978) p. 197-202.

93. Vela C., Platas C., Gurbindo C., Tricas L., Subiza E., Garcia R. and Lahoz C.
Fractionation and biological characterization of Olea europea pollen extract. Int Archs Allergy appl Immunol 68 (1982) p. 289-294.

94. Rakoski J. a nd Düngemann H.
Kreuzsensibilisierung bei Pollen von Compositen (Asteraceae) − Untersuchungen mit PRICK-Test, RAST und RAST-Inhibitionstest. Z Hautkr 55 (1980):11 p. 741-747.

95. Mulder J. and Verhaar M.A.T.
In vitro screening of allergy by mixed allergen extracts. Ircs-Biochem 8 (1980) p. 221.

96. Kern F., Sobotka A.K., Valentine M .D., Benton A.W. and Lichtenstein L.M.
Allergy to insect sting. III. Allergenic cross-reactivity among the vespid venoms. J Allergy Clin Immunol 57 (1976) p. 554-559.

97. Ahlstedt S., Eriksson N., Lindgren S. and Roth A.
Specific IgE determination by RAST compared with skin and provocation tests in allergy diagnosis with birch pollen, timothy pollen and dog epithelium allergens. Clin Allergy 4 (1974) p. 131-140.

98. Apold J.
RAST (Radio-Allergo-Sorbent-Test) i Klinisk Allergidiagnostik. Tidsskr Nor Lägeforen 94 (1974) p. 918-922.

99. Al-Tikriti S.K., Al-Salihi M. and Gaillard G.E.
Pollen and mold survey of Baghdad, Iraq. Ann Allergy 45 (1980) p. 97-99.

100. Müller U., Reisman R., Wypych J., Elliott W., Steger R., Walsh S. and Arbesman C.
Comparison of vespid venoms collected by electrostimulation and by sac extraction. J Allergy Clin Immunol 68 (1981) p. 254-261.

101. Yman L., Ponterius G. and Brandt R.
RAST -based allergen assay methods. Dev Biol Stand 29 (1975) p. 151-165.

102. Kleinhans D.
Allergenspezifisches Immunoglobulin E im Serum (RAST), Hauttests und konjunktivale provokationstests mit häufigen pollen-allergenen bei Pollinose-patienten. Z Hautkr 51 (1976) p. 609-616.

103. Brückner V., Noster U., Schulz K.H. and Stute J.
Beziehung zwischen Hauttest und spezifischem IgE (Radio-Allergo-Sorbent-Test) in der Diagnostik inhalativer Allergien. Z Hautkr 52 (1977) p. 109-116.

104. Varga J.M. and Ceska M.
Characterization of allergen extracts by gel isoelectrofocusing and radioimmunosorbent allergen assay. Allergens in timothy pollen (Phleum pratense) extracts. J Allergy Clin Immunol 49 (1972) p. 274-284.

105. Foucard T.
A follow-up study of children with asthmatoid bronchitis I. Skin test reactions and IgE antibodies to common allergens. Acta Paediatr Scand 62 (1973) p. 633-644.

106. Foucard T., Bennich H. and Johansson S.G.O.
Studies on the stability of diluted allergen extracts using the radioallergosorbent test (RAST). Clin Allergy 3 (1973) p. 91-102.

107. Wüthrich B.
Allergen-spezifische IgE im Radio-allergo-sorbent-test bei Neur odermitis. Hautarzt 25 (1974) p. 603-605.

108. Havenen J., Apold H., Hvatum M., Oseid S. and Aas K.
The radioallergosorbent test in the in vitro diagnosis of multiple reaginic allergy. Comparison of two different extract preparations, from timothy pollen, birch pollen and dog's hair, respectively as used for tests in vivo and in vitro. Clin Allergy 4 (1974) p. 411-420.

109. Weeke B., Løwenstein H. and Nielsen L.
Allergens in timothy pollen identified by crossed-radio-immuno-electrophoresis (CRIE). Acta Allergol 29 (1974) p. 402-417.

110. Hoffman D.R. and McDonald C.A.
Allergens in Hymenoptera venom. XI. Species specificity to Polistes (paper wasp) venoms. Ann Allergy 48 (1982) p. 82-88.

111. Torres-Rodriques J.M.
Comparison between total and specific IgE with intradermal testing in human hydatidosis. Proc 12th Congress of the European Academy of Allergology and Clin Immunology, Rome Vol XXX, Supp 4 1983, p. 75.

112. Wypych J.I., Reisman R.E., Elliott W.B., Steger R.J. and Arbesman C.E.
Immunologic and biochemical evaluation of the potency of whole insect body extracts. J Allergy Clin Immunol 63 (1979) p. 267-272.

113. Weeke E., Løwenstein H., Prahl P. and Weeke B.
Värdien af radioallergosorbentteknik (RAST) i Diagnosen af asthma bronchiale hos børn. Ugeskr Laeg 138 (1976) p. 2712-2717.

114. Hunt K.J., Sobotka A.K., Valentine M.D., Yunginger J.W. and Lichtenstein L.M.
Sensitization following Hymenoptera whole body extract therapy. J Allergy Clin Immunol 61 (1978) p. 48-53.

115. Kleinhans D.
Der Radio-Allergo-Sorbens-Test
(RAST) zur ermittlung der Bienenallergie
von soforttyp. Vortrag: 31. Tagung
Deutsche Dermat. Gesell. Köln,
April 2nd, 1977.

116. Osterhage F., Wippler M., Kallden J.R.
and Deicher H.
Determination of specific IgE and IgG
serum antibodies during immunotherapy in hay fever patients by RAST. Z
Immunitätsforsch 153 (1977) p. 189-
203.

117. Light W.C., Reisman R.E., Rosario N.A.
and Arbesman C.E.
Comparison of the allergenic properties
of bee venom and whole bee body
extract. Clin Allergy 6 (1976)
p. 293-300.

118. Kjellman N.I.M., Lanner Å. and Roth A.
Predictive value of serum IgE levels
during rush hyposensitization. Clin
Allergy (1977) p. 465-471.

119. Frostad A.B., Bolle R., Grimmer O.E.
and Aas K.
A new well-characterized, purified
allergen preparation from timothy
pollen. II. Allergenic in vivo and in vitro
properties. Int Arch Allergy appl
Immunol 55 (1977) p. 35-40.

120. Grimmer O.E., Bolle R., Frostad A.
and Aas K.
A new well-characerized, purified
allergen preparation from timothy
pollen. III. Immunological properties in
the human immunoglobulin E system.
Int Arch Allergy appl Immunol 55 (1977)
p. 41-46.

121. Eriksson N.E. and Ahlstedt S.
Diagnosis of reaginic allergy with house
dust, animal dander and pollen
allergens in adult patients. V. A comparison between the enzyme linked
immunosorbent assay (ELISA), provocation tests, skin tests and RAST.
Int Arch Allergy appl Immunol 54 (1977)
p. 88-95.

122. Barnard J.H.
Studies of 400 Hymenoptera sting
deaths in the United States. J Allergy
Clin Immunol 52 (1973) p. 259-264.

123. Eriksson N.E.
Food sensitivity reported by patients
with asthma and hay fever. Allergy 33
(1978) p. 189-196.

124. Barr S.E.
Allergy to Hymenoptera stings – review
of the world literature: 1953-19 70.
Ann Allergy 29 (1971) p. 49-66.

125. Witassek F.
Nachweis von total und spezifischen
IgE bei Patienten mit Echinokokkose.
Gemeinsame Fagung der Deutschen
Tropenmedizinschen Gesellschaft
Österreicheschen und Schweize-
reischen Gesellschaft für
Tropenmedizin und Parasitologie in
Garmisch-Partenkirchen, 22 April,
1983. Abstract 78

126. Löscher Th.
Der Radioallergosorbenttest (RAST) in
der Diagnostik und Therapiekontrolle
der Echinokokkose. Ibid, Abstract 80.

127. Parrish H.M.
Analysis of 400 fatalities from
venomous animals in the United States.
Am J Med Sci (1963) p. 129-141.

128. Relyveld E.H. and Henocq E.
Analysis and standardization of allergen
extracts intended for therapeutic use.
Allergy 35 (1980) p. 218-220.

129. Schröder H. and Yman L.
Standardization of the RAST inhibition
assay. Allergy 35 (1980) p. 234-236.

130. Leupold W., Wunderlich P., Schollberg
K. and Mittenzwey K.W.
Bedeutung des Radio-Allergo-Sorbent-
Tests (RAST) in der allergologischen
Diagnostik des Asthma bronchiale im
Kindesalter. Kinderärztl Prax 48 (1980)
p. 98-102.

131. Jarisch R.
Die Bienengiftallergie (modell einer IgE-mediierten soforttypallergie). Wien Klin Wochenschr 92 (1980) Suppl 122, p. 2-27.

132. Österballe O., Løwenstein H., Prahl O., Skov P. and Weeke B.
Immunotherapy in hay fever with two major allergens 19, 25 and partially purified extract of timothy grass pollen. Allergy 36 (1981) p. 183-199.

133. Data on file. Comparison of Phadebas RAST® discs g5 and g7.

134. Lundkvist U.
Research and development of the RAST technology. Advances in diagnosis of allergy: RAST. Proc 1st N. Amer Conf. on RAST, Palm Springs, Ca. 1975 Ed. by R Evans III. Miami, Fla. (Symposia Specialists) 1975. p. 85-99.

135. Müller U., Thurnheer U., Patrizzi R., Spiess J. and Hoigne R.
Immunotherapy in bee sting hypersensitivity. Bee venom versus whole body extract. Allergy 34 (1979) p. 369-378.

136. Grant J., Rahr R., Rhueson D., Gold blum R. and Lett-Brown M.
Diagnosis and treatment with wasp venom. Adv Allergol appl Immunol Congr Jerusalem 1979 p. 435-440.

137. Settipane G.A. and Carlisle C.C.
A critical evaluation of RAST to venoms of Hymenoptera. Clin Allergy 10 (1980) p. 667-673.

138. Spath P., Huber H., Ludvan M., Roth A., Schwarz S. and Zelger J.
Determinations of penicilloyl specific IgE antibodies for the evaluation of hypersensitivity against penicillin. Allergy 34 (1979) p. 405-411.

139. Koivikko A.
Patient exposure to moulds. Paper presented at the Mould Allergy Workshop, Uppsala, Sweden, September 23, 1983.

140. Kang B.
Study on cockroach antigen as a probable causative agent in bronchial asthma. J Allergy Clin Immunol 58 (1976) p. 357-365.

141. Mathur S., Goust J-M. Horger E.O. and Fudenberg H.H.
Immunoglobulin E anti-Candida antibodies and candidiasis. Infection and Immunity Oct (1977) p. 257-259.

142. Twarog F.J., Picone F.J., Strunk R.S., So J. and Colten H.R.
Immediate hypersensitivity to cockroach. Isolation and purification of the major antigens. J Allergy Clin Immunol 59 (1977) p. 154-160.

143. Baldo B.A., Krilis S. and Wrigley C.W.
Hypersensitivity to inhaled flour allergens. Comparison between cereals. Allergy 35 (1980) p. 45-56.

144. Anfosso F., Soler M., Mallea M. and Charpin J.
Isolation and characterization in vitro of an allergen from plane-tree (Platanus acerifolia) pollen. Int Archs Allergy appl Immun 54 (1977) p. 481-486.

145. Yoo T.J., Kuo C.Y. and Joseph S.
Induction of anti-timothy pollen reaginic antibodies and their cross reactivity in the rat. Ann Allergy 39 (1977) p. 272-275.

146. Data on file G48. Kjellman M. Specific IgE determinations in patients with hypersensitivity to pollen from Holcus lanatus and Secale cerealae. Nov, 1980.

147. Kalveram K.J. and Forck G.
Cross-reactivity between grass and corn pollen antigens. Int Archs Allergy appl Immunol 57 (1978) p. 549-553.

148. Olenchock S.A., Mull J.C. and Major P.C.
Complement activation by commercial allergen extracts of cereal grains. Clin Allergy 10 (1980) p. 395-404.

149. Perera M.G., Bernstein I.L., Michael J.G. and Johansson S.G.O.
Predictability of the radioallergosorbent test (RAST) in ragweed pollinosis. Am Rev Respir Dis 111 (1975) p. 605-610.

150. Kang B. and Sulit N.
A comparative study of prevalence of skin hypersensitivity to cockroach and house dust antigens. Ann Allergy 41 (1978) p. 333-336.

151. Rosedale N. and Browne K.
Hyposensitisation in the management of recurring vaginal candidiasis. Ann Allergy 43 (1979) p. 250-253.

152. Ito K., Sano Y., Okudaira H., Morita H., Nakagawa T., Sakamoto Y. and Miyamoto T.
Studies on relation between skin reaction and RAST score using Candida and Cedar discs. Arerogi no Rinshi (Trans. Clin Allergol) 17 (1982) p. 59-64 (Japan, Eng. abstract).

153. Morita Y., Miyamoto T., Horiuchi Y., Oshima S., Katsuhata S. and Kawal S.
Further studies in allergenic identity between house dust and the house dust mite, Dermatophagoides farinae Hughes, 1961. Ann Allergy 35 (1975) p. 361-366.

154. Kino T. and Oshima S.
Radioallergosorbent test (RAST) on fungal allergens in patients with bronchial asthma, with special reference to Candida RAST and the accuracy of its measurement. Clin Immunol 14 (1982):10 p.906-916. (Japan. English abstract).

155. Hoffman D.R.
Comparison of methods of performing the radioallergosorbent test: Phadebas, Fadal-Nalebuff and Hoffman protocols. Ann Allergy 45 (1980) p. 343-346.

156. Hulett A.C. and Dockhorn R.J.
House dust, mite (D.farinae) and cockroach allergy in a midwestern population. Ann Allergy 42 (1979) p. 160-165.

157. Goodfriend L., Roebber M., Lundkvist U. and Choudhury A.M
Two variants of ragweed allergen ra3. J Allergy Clin Immunol 67 (1981) p. 299-304.

158. Data on file. Comparison of cow sera and cow dander.

159. King T.P.
Immunochemical studies of ragweed pollen allergens. Allergy 35 (1980) p. 187-211.

160. Yunginger J.W. and Gleich G.J.
Measurement of ragweed antigen E by a double antibody radioimmunoassay. J Allergy Clin Immunol 59 (1972) p. 326-337.

161. Virchow C., Roth A., Debelić M. and Möller E.
Vergleich zwischen RAST und In-vivo Tests in der Diagnostik von Compositenpollen-Sensibilisierung. Prax Pneumol 30 (1976) p. 11-18.

162. Adkinson N.F. Jr.
Recent developments in the use of RAST for determining hypersensitivity to penicillin. In: Adv in Diagnosis of Allergy: RAST (ed: Evans R III) Symposia Specialists, Miami (1975) p. 125-136.

163. Bayer A.S., Blumenkrantz M.J., Montgomerie J.Z., Galpin J.E., Coburn J.W. and Guze L.B.
Candida peritonitis. Report of 22 cases and review of the English literature. Am J Med 61 (1976) p. 832-840.

164. Berger M., Kirkpatrick C.H., Goldstein P.K. and Gallin J.I.
IgE antibodies to Staphylococcus aureus and Candida albicans in patients with the syndrome of hyper-immunoglobulin E and recurrent effects. J Immunol 125 (1980) p. 2437-2447.

165. Koranda W. and Pfeifer R.
Bedeutung von Hauttest und RAST für die Diagnostik der Insektenstichallergie. Wien Med Wochenschr 131 (1981) p. 301-303.

166. *Juhlin L. and Wide L.*
IgE antibodies and pencillin allergy.
Mechanisms in Drug Allergy (ed: Dash,
C.H. Jones, H E H). Churchill
Livingstone, Edinburg and London
(1972) p. 139.

167. *Eriksson N.E.*
Allergy to pollen from different
deciduous trees in Sweden. An
investigation with skin tests,
provocation tests and the
Radioallergosorbent test (RAST) in
springtime hay fever patients. Allergy 33
(1978) p. 299-309.

168. *Yman L., Roosdorp N., Schröder H.
and Andrae M-L.*
Methods for the determination of IgE
and allergen-specific antibodies. Int
Allergy Symp., Uppsala, 24-26 Sept.,
1980, p. 74-83.

169. *Hill H.R.*
The syndrome of hyperimmuno-
globulinemia E and recurrent infections.
Am J Dis Child 136 (1982) p. 767-771.

170. *Wide L. and Juhlin L.*
Detection of penicillin allergy of the
immediate type by radioimmunoassay
of reagine (IgE) to pencilloyl conjugates.
Clin Allergy 1 (1971) p. 171-177.

171. *Tovey E. and Vandenberg R.*
Mite allergen content in commercial
extracts and in bed dust determined by
radioallergosorbent test. Clin Allergy 9
(1979) p. 253-262.

172. *Urbanek R.*
Hausstaub und Hausstaubmilbe.
Arb Paul Ehrlich Inst Georg Speyer
Haus Ferdinand Blum Inst 73 (1978)
p. 126-134.

173. *Patrizzi R., Müller U., Yman L.
and Hoigné R.*
Comparison of skin test and RAST
for the diagnosis of bee sting allergy.
Allergy 34 (1979) p. 249-256.

174. *Kurvits J.*
Verbesserte RAST-Methode durch
Einführung eines neuen Anti-IgE (D_ε2).
RAST 2 Berichtsband (1981) p. 1-5
(Grosse Verlag) 1981.

175. *Arsdel van P.P., O'Rourke T.K.,
Horan J.D. and Kumasaka Y.*
Serum haemagglutinating antibodies in
penicillin allergy. JAMA 185 (1963)
p. 584.

176. *Aalberse R.C.*
Allergens in house dust. Acta Oto-
Rhino-Laryngol Belg 32 (1978)
p. 25-31.

177. *King T.P., Sobotka A.K., Alagon A.,
Kochoumian L. and Lichtenstein L.M.*
Protein allergens of white-faced
hornet, yellow hornet, and yellow jacket
venoms. Biochemistry 17 (1978)
p. 5165-5174.

178. *Weck de A.L.*
Low molecular weight antigens. In: The
antigens. Sela M (ed) Academic Press,
New York 2 (1974) p. 141.

179. *Müller U., Roth A., Yman L.
and Patrizzi R.*
Use of RAST technique in wasp sting
hypersensitivity. Cross-reactions
between various insect antigens are
specially considered. Allergy 33 (1978)
p. 197-202.

180. *Sachs N.I., Joves R.T. and Yunginger
J.W.*
Isolation and partial characterization of
a major peanut allergen. J Allergy Clin
Immunol 67 (1981) p. 27-34.

181. *Derrick E.*
Relative importance of various plants
in causation of hay fever and asthma
in Australia. Med J Aust 1 (1962)
p. 972-977.

182. *Baldo B.A., Sutton R. and Wrigley C.W.*
Grass allergens with particular
reference to cereals. Prog Allergy 30
p. 1-66 (Karger, Basel 1982).

183. *Bryant D.H. and Burns M.W.*
Skin prick test reactions to inhalant
allergens in asthmatic patients.
Med J Aust 1 (1976) p. 918-924.

184. *Baldo B.A., Chensee Q.J., Howden
M.E.H. and Sharp P.J.*
Allergens from plantain (*Plantago
lanceolata*). Studies with pollen
extracts. Int Archs Allergy appl Immunol
68 (1982) p. 295-304.

185. Drug Ther Bull – Penicillin Allergy 13
(1975):3.

186. *Hoffman D.R.*
The use and interpretation of RAST to
stinging insect venoms. Ann Allergy 42
(1979) p. 224-230.

187. *Selcow J.E., Mendelson L.M. and
Rosen J.P.*
Anaphylactic reactions in skin test-
negative patients. J Allergy Clin
Immunol 65 (1980) p. 400.

188. *Dewdney J.M.*
Immunology of the antibodies. In: The
antigens. Sela M (ed) Academic Press,
New York 4 (1977) p. 74-245.

189. *Hoffman D.R.*
Allergens in *Hymenoptera* venom. VI.
Cross-reactivity of human IgE
antibodies to the three vespid venoms
and between vespid and paper wasp
venoms. Ann Allergy 46 (1981)
p. 304-309.

190. *Newmark F.M.*
The hay fever plants of Colorado. Ann
Allergy 40 (1978) p. 18.

191. *Shafiee A., Yunginger J.W. and
Gleich G.J.*
Isolation and characterization of
Russian thistle (*Salsola pestifer*) pollen
allergens. J Allergy Clin Immunol 67
(1981) p. 472-481.

192. *Spieksma F.T.M., Charpin H., Nolard D.
and Stix E.*
City spore concentrations in the
European economic community (EEC).
IV. Summer weed pollen (*Rumex,
Plantago, Chenopodiaceae, Artemisia*),
1976 and 1977. Clin Allergy 10 (1980)
p. 319-329.

193. *Solomon W.R.*
An appraisal of *Rumex* pollen as an
aeroallergen. J Allergy 44 (1969) p. 25.

194. *Wagatsuma Y. and Matsuyama T.*
Pollinosis by *Rumex acetosella* (sheep
sorrel) and *Rumex obtusifolius* (blunt-
leaved dock). Japanese J Allergy 23
(1974) p. 23.

195. *Panzani R.*
L'asthme pollinique á la Parietarie.
Presse Medicale 64 (1956) p. 908.

196. *Serafini U.*
Studies on hay fever (with special
regard to pollinosis due to *Parietaria
officinalis*). Acta Allergologica 11 (1975)
p. 3.

197. Data on file G55. Personnal
communication to Pharmacia from P.
Calderón G., André Bigaux S.A.,
Division Diagnostica, Coyoacán,
Mexico, November 1983.

198. *Weeke E.R., Jørgensen G., Petersen
B.N., Torp U. and Buch H.*
Pollenregistrering i København
sommaren 1977. Ugeskr Laeg 141
(1979) p. 1194-1199.

199. *Horak F., Hussarek M., Jäger S.
and Skoda-Türk R.*
Die Bestimmung der Aggressivität
allergisierender Pollenarten. Wien Klin
Wochenschr 92 (1980) p. 161-164.

200. *Belin L.*
Immunological analysis of birch pollen
antigens with special reference to the
allergenic components. Int Arch Allergy
42 (1972) p. 300.

201. Wüthrich B. and Kopper E.
Nachweis von Spezifischen IgE-
Serumantikörpern mit dem Radio-
Allergo-Sorbent-Test (RAST) und seine
Bedeutung für die Diagnostik der
atopischen Allergie. Schweiz Med
Wochenschr 105 (1975) p. 1337-1345.

202. Ahlstedt S., Ekström B., Svärd P.O.,
Sjöberg B., Kristofferson A. and
Örtengren B.
New aspects on antigens in penicillin
allergy. CRC Crit Rev Toxicol 1 (1980)
p. 219.

203. Eriksson N.E., Ahlstedt S. and
Løvhagen O.
Immunotherapy in spring-time hay
fever. A clinical and immunological
study comparing two different
treatment extract compositions.
Allergy 34 (1979) p. 233-247.

204. Dhorranintra B. and Bunnag C.
Cross reactions in skin tests between
kapok and house dust allergenic
extracts. Ann Allergy 39 (1977)
p. 201-203.

205. Shapiro S., Slone D., Siskind V.
and Lewis G.P.
Drug rash with ampicillin and other
penicillin. Lancet 2 (1969).

206. Bessot J.C., Ott W., Thierry R. and
Pauli G.
Allergie aux pollens d'arbres en Alsace.
II. Apport du RAST direct et de
l'inhibition du RAST a l'identification
des allergènes responsables. Rev
Fr Allergol 21 (1981) p. 7-12.

207. Bronswijk von J.E.M.H. and Rijckärt G.
Hausstaubbiologie als hilfe
bei der Hausstauballergieprohylaxe.
Therapiewoche 30 (1980)
p. 6161-6164.

208. Diagnosis and treatment of IgE-
mediated diseases. Ed.: SGO
Johansson Excerpta Medica,
Amsterdam, 1981, p. 74.

209. Biliotti G., Romagnani S. and Ricci M.
Mites and house dust allergy. IV.
Antigen and allergen(s) of Dermato-
phagoides pteronyssinus extract. Clin
Allergy (1975:1) p. 69-77.

210. Maunsell K., Wraith D.G. and
Hughes A.M.
Hyposensitization in mite asthma.
Lancet (1971:1) p. 967-968.

211. Voorhorst R.
The human dander atopy. II. Human
dander, a complicating factor in the
study of the relationship between house
dust and Dermatophagoides allergens.
Ann Allergy 39 (1977) p. 339-343.

212. Brighton W.D., and Topping M.D.
Human dander in house dust allergy.
Clin Allergy 7 (1977) p. 577-582.

213. Chaikovsky V.T., Sosnkin I.E. and
Mirzoyan I.M.
Occupational dermatoses in workers
of meat packing plants. Vestnik
Dermatologii i venerologii (USSR) 47
(1973) p. 76-78.

214. Collins-Williams C., Hung F. and
Bremner K.
House dust mite and house dust
allergy. Ann Allergy 37 (1976) p. 12-17.

215. Berrens L.
The allergens in house dust. Progr
Allergy 14 (1970) p. 259-339.

216. Viander M., Fräki J., Djupsund B.M. and
Laine S.
Antigens and allergens in birch pollen
extract. Allergy 34 (1979) p. 289-302.

217. Puttonen E. and Pilström L.
Purification of birch pollen allergen
extract by gel filtration. I. Chemical and
immunological characterization of the
fractions. Int Arch Allergy appl Immunol
61 (1980) p. 299-307.

218. Björksten F., Halmepuro L.,
Hannuksela M. and Lahti A.
Extraction and properties of apple
allergens. Allergy 35 (1980) p. 671-677.

219. Pauli G., Bessot J.C., Thierry R. and
Lamensans A.
Correlation between skin tests,
inhalation tests and specific IgE in a
study of 120 subjects allergic to house
dust and Dermatophagoides
pteronyssinus. Clin Allergy 7 (1977)
p. 337-346.

220. *Apold J., Florvaag E. and Elsayed S.*
Comparative studies on tree-pollen allergens. I. Isolation and partial characterization of a major allergen from birch pollen (*Betula verrucosa*). Int Arch Allergy appl Immunol 64 (1981) p. 439-447.

221. *Tuft L. and Heck V.M.*
Mites as antigenic excitants of house dust allergy: Report of some allergy studies. Ann Allergy 33 (1974) p. 325-330.

222. *Blythe M.E.*
Some aspects of the ecological study of the house dust mites. Br J Dis Chest 70 (1976) p. 3.

223. *Henson G.E.*
Garlic: an occupational factor in the etiology of bronchial asthma. J Fla Med Assoc 27 (1940) p. 86.

224. *Lybarger J.A., Gallagher J.S., Pulver D.W., Litwin A., Brooks S. and Bernstein I.L.*
Occupational asthma induced by inhalation and ingestion of garlic. J Allergy Clin Immunol 69 (1982) p. 448-454

225. *Maunsell K., Wraith D .G. and Cunnington A.M.*
Mites and house dust allergy in bronchial asthma. Lancet 1 (1968) p. 1267.

226. *Voorhorst R., Spieksma-Boezman M.I.A. and Spieksma F.T.M.*
Is a mite (D.sp.) the producer of the house dust allergen. Allergic Asthma 10 (1964) p. 329.

227. *Dekker H.*
Asthma and mites. Münch Med Wschr 75 (1928) p. 515.

228. *Yoo T.J., Spitz E. and McGerit y J.L.*
Conifer pollen allergy: Studies of immunogenicity and cross antigenicity of conifer pollens in rabbit and man. Ann Allergy 34 (1975) p. 87-93.

229. *Glaubitt D., Mühlenberg R. and Siafarikas K.*
Die komplementaere Bedeutung von Radio-Allergo Sorbens-Tests in der Diagnostik von Allergien gegen Hausstaub und Milben bei Kindern. Z Hautkr 54 (1979) p. 287-294.

230. *Mansfield L.E. and Nelson H.S.*
Allergens in commercial house dust. Ann Allergy 48 (1982) p. 205-209.

231. *Bousquet J., Hale R., Guerin B. and Michel F.B.*
Enzymatic activities of house dust extracts. Ann Allergy 45 (1980) p. 316-321.

232. *Zetterström O., Fagerberg E. and Wide L.*
An investigation of pollen extracts from different deciduous trees in patients with springtime allergy in Sweden. Acta Allergol 27 (1972) p. 15-21.

233. Data on file G55. Screening for positive hamster sera among positive guinea pig sera.

234. *Hoffman D.R. and Haddad Z.H.*
Diagnosis of multiple inhalant allergies in children by radio-immunoassay. Pediatrics 54 (1974) p. 151-156.

235. *Cernelc S.*
Relationship between the house dust and mite allergen by immunochemical and clinical evidence. Allerg Immunol 26 (1980) p. 31-40.

236. *Berrens L., Bruynzeel P.L.B., Fradkin V.A., Henocq E., Hoek G.T., Kersten W., Lavrenchik E.I. and Petrunov B.*
Purification and standardization of house dust allergens based on cutaneous tests, RAST-inhibition, and complement assay. Allergy 35 (1980) p. 222-224.

237. *Wüthrich B. and Annen H.*
Pollinosis: I. Ermittlungen zur Klinik und zum Pollenspektrum an 1565 Pollenallergikern. Schweiz Med Wochenschr 109 (1979) p. 1212-1218.

238. *Yunginger J.W., Jones R.T., Nesheim M.E. and Geller M.*
Studies on *Alternaria* allergens. III. Isolation of a major allergenic fraction (Alt-II). J Allergy Clin Immunol 66 (1980) p. 138-147.

239. *Merrett T.G., Pantin C.F.A., Dimond A.H. and Merrett J.*
Screening for IgE-mediated allergy. Allergy 35 (1980) p. 491-501.

240. *Vijay H.M., Huang H., Young N.M and Bernstein I.L.*
Studies on *Alternaria* allergens. I. Isolation of allergens from *Alternaria tenuis* and *Alternaria solani*. Int Arch Allergy appl Immunol 60 (1979) p. 229-239.

241. *Langeland T.*
A clinical and immunological study of allergy to hen's egg white. Allergy 38 (1983) p. 493-500.

242. *Falleroni A.E., Zeiss R. and Levitz D.*
Occupational asthma secondary to inhalation of garlic dust. J Allergy Clin Immunol 68 (1981) p. 156-160.

243. *Yunginger J.W., Roberts G.D. and Gleich G.J.*
Studies on *Alternaria* allergens. I. Establishment of the radioallergo-sorbent test for measurement of *Alternaria* allergens. J Allergy Clin Immunol 57 (1976) p. 293-301.

244. *Saito Y., Hasegawa M . and Arrendal H.*
Evaluation of radio-allergo-sorbent test for diagnosis of Japanese cedar pollinosis. 2nd Int Symp Infection and Allergy of the nose and paranasal sinuses, Bologna, Italy, October 20-23, 1980.

245. *Horiguti S. and Saito Y.*
Clinical observations on hay fever due to Japanese cedar pollen. Bull Tokyo Med Dent Univ 14 (1967) p. 141-155.

246. *Saito Y.*
Aerobiological and clinical studies on allergenic pollens in Tokyo area. Bull Tokyo Med Dent Univ 18 (1971) p. 95-104.

247. *Takayma S., Saito Y., Watanabe K. and Hasegawa M.*
In vitro analysis of Japanese Cedar pollinosis with radioimmunosorbent test and radioallergosorbent test. Proc International Symposium of Infection and Allergy of the Nose and paranasal sinuses, Tokyo, 1976, p. 98-102.

248. *Mogi G., Maeda S., Yoshida T. and Watanabe N.*
IgE studies on respiratory tract allergies. Arch Otolaryngol 103 (1977) p. 251-257.

249. *Hausen B.M. and Schmalle H.*
Quinonoid constituents as contact sensitisers in Australian blackwood (*Acacia melanoxylon* RBR). Br J Ind Med 38 (1981) p. 105-109.

250. *Novey H.S., Roth M. and Wells I.D.*
Mesquite pollen — an aeroallergen in asthma and allergic rhinitis. J Allergy Clin Immunol 59 (1977) p. 359-363.

251. *Singh A.B. and Babu C.R.*
Studies on pollen allergy in Delhi. Allergy 35 (1980) p. 311-317.

252. *Singh A.B. and Babu C.R.*
Survey of atmospheric pollen allergens in Delhi: seasonal periodicity. Ann Allergy 48 (1982) p. 115-122.

253. *Yunginger J.W., Jones R.T. and Gleich G.J.*
Studies on *Alternaria* allergens. II. Measurement of the relative potency of commercial *Alternaria* extracts by the direct RAST and by RAST inhibition. J Allergy Clin Immunol 58 (1976) p. 405-413.

254. *Elsayed S. and Apold J.*
Immunochemical analysis of cod fish allergen M: Locations of the immuno-globulin binding sites as demonstrated by the native and synthetic peptides. Allergy 38 (1983) p. 449-459.

255. *Aas K.*
The diagnosis of hypersensitivity to ingested foods. Reliability of skin prick testing and the radioallergosorbent test with different materials. Clin Allergy 8 (1978) p. 39-50.

256. Gavani U.D., Hyde J.S. and Moore B.S.
Hypersensitivity to milk and egg white.
Skin tests, RAST results and clinical
intolerance. Ann Allergy 40 (1978)
p. 314-318.

257. Schumacher M.J., McClatchy J.K.,
Farr R.S. and Minden P.
Primary interaction between antibody
and components of Alternaria. I.
Immunological and chemical
characteristics of labelled antigens.
J Allergy Clin Immunol 56 (1975)
p. 39-53.

258. Hoffman D.R. and Haddad Z.H.
Diagnosis of IgE-mediated reactions to
food antigens by radioimmunoassay.
J Allergy Clin Immunol 54 (1974)
p. 165-173.

259. Data on file G55. Comparison of
allergens in polished and unpolished
rice.

260. Dopico G.A., Flaherty D., Bhansali P.
and Chavaje N.
Grain fever syndrome induced
by inhalation of airborne grain dust.
J Allergy Clin Immunol 69 (1982)
p. 435-443.

261. Mühlenberg R., Glaubitt D., Siafarikas
K. and Staude E.
Radioallergosorbent-tests bei Kindern.
Nuklearmediziner 1 (1978) p. 159-164.

262. Lessof M.H., Wraith D.G., Merret T.G.,
Buisseret P.D. Merrett J.
Food allergy and intolerance in 100
patients – local and systemic effects.
Q J Med 49 (1980) p. 259-271.

263. Rijckärt G. and Broers J.I.V.
Time dependent release of allergens
from some xerophilic fungi. Allergy 35
(1980) p. 679-682.

264. Aukrust L., Almeland T., Refsum D.
and Aas K.
Severe hypersensitivity of intolerance
reactions to measles vaccine in six
children. Allergy 35 (1980) p. 581-587.

265. Jones D.B., Kerr G.D., Parker J.H.
and Wilson R.S.E.
Dietary allergy and specific IgE
in ulcerative colitis. J R Soc Med 74
(1981) p. 292-293.

266. Björksten F. and Saarinen U.M.
IgE antibodies to cow's milk in infants
fed breast milk and milk formulae.
Lancet (1978:2) p. 624-625.

267. Saarinen U.M., Björskten F., Knekt P.
and Siimes M.A.
Serum immunoglobulin E in healthy
infants fed breast milk or cow's milk-
based formulae. Clin Allergy 9 (1979)
p. 339-345.

268. Haddad Z.H., Kalra V. and Verma S.
IgE antibodies to peptic and peptic-
tryptic digests of betalactoglobulin:
Significance in food hypersensitivity.
Ann Allergy 42 (1979) p. 368-371.

269. Dannaeus A. and Johansson S.G.O.
A follow-up study of infants with
adverse reactions to cow's milk. I.
Serum IgE, skin test reactions and
RAST in relation to clinical course. Acta
Paediatr Scand 68 (1979) p. 377-382.

270. Fällström S.P., Ahlstedt S. and
Hanson L.A.A.
Specific antibodies in infants with
gastrointestinal intolerance to cow's
milk protein. Int Arch Allergy appl
Immunol 56 (1978) p. 97-105.

271. Kauffmann H.F. and de Vries K.
Antibodies against Aspergillus
fumigatus. II. Idenfication and
quantification by means of crossed
immunoelectrophoresis. Int Arch Allergy
appl Immunol 62 (1980) p. 265-275.

272. Hattevig G., Kjellman B.,
Johansson SGO. and Björkstén B.
Clinical symptoms and IgE responses
to common food proteins in atopic and
healthy children. In press, 1984.

273. Kauffman H.F. and de Vries K.
Antibodies against Aspergillus
fumigatus. I. Standardization of the
antigenic composition. Int Arch Allergy
appl Immunol 62 (1980) p. 252-264.

274. Kjellman N.I.M. and Johansson S.G.O.
Soy versus cow's milk in infants with a
biparental history of atopic disease:
Development of atopic disease and
immunoglobulins from birth to 4 years
of age. Clin Allergy 9 (1979) p. 347-358.

275. Mackie R.M., Cobb S.J., Cochran R.E.I.
and Thomson J.
Total and specific IgE levels in patients
with atopic dermatitis. The correlation
between prick testing, clinical history of
allergy, and in vitro quantification of IgE
during clinical exacerbation and
remission. Clin Exp Dermatol 4 (1979)
p. 187-195.

276. Kim S.J. and Chaparas S.D.
Characterization of antigens from
Aspergillus fumigatus. III. Comparison
of antigenitic relationships of clinically
important aspergilli. Am Rev Respir
Dis 120 (1979) p. 1297-1303.

277. Slavin R.G.
What does a fungus among us really
mean? J Allergy Clin Immunol 62 (1978)
p. 7-8.

278. Juto P. and Björksten B.
Serum IgE in infants and influence of
type of feeding. Clin Allergy 10 (1980)
p. 593-600.

279. Endre L., Osváth P. and Péter F.
Untersuchung des IgE-Spiegels Milch-
und Eierantigenspezifischer Sera bei
allergischen Kindern. Allerg Immunol 26
(1980) p. 15-20.

280. Weiss N., Speiser F. and Hussain R.
IgE antibodies in human
onchocerciasis. Application of a
newly developed radioallergosorbent
test (RAST). Acta Tropica (1981)
p. 353-362.

281. Data on file G55. Comparison of
A.plantanoides and A.negundo RAST®
discs.

282. Flaherty D.K., Murray H.D. and
Reed C.E.
Cross reactions to antigens causing
hypersensitivity pneumonitis. J Allergy
Clin Immunol 53 (1974) p. 329-335.

283. Firer M.A., Hosking C.S. and Hill D.J.
Effect of antigen load on development
of milk antibodies in infants allergic to
milk. Br Med J 283 (1981) p. 693-695.

284. Schwartz H.R., Nerurkar L.S., Spies
J.R., Scanlon R.T. and Bellanti J.A.
Milk hypersensitivity: RAST studies
using new antigens generated by
pepsin hydrolysis of beta-lactoglobulin.
Ann Allergy 45 (1980) p. 242-245.

285. Aas K. and Lundkvist U.
The radioallergosorbent test with a
purified allergen from codfish. Clin
Allergy 3 (1973) p. 255-261.

286. Lahti A.., Björkstén F. and
Hannuksela M.
Allergy to birch pollen and apple and
cross-reactivity of the allergens
studied with RAST. Allergy 35 (1980)
p. 297-300.

287. McCarthy D.S. and Pepys J.
Pulmonary aspergilloma – clinical
immunology. Clin Allergy 3 (1973)
p. 57-70.

288. Sergyels R. and Michel O.
Asthme et candidose. Les traitements
hyposensibilisants. Ed. Y. Robience.
Symp. Nov 1983, HALAB Allergy
Service, Belgium.

289. Müller R., de Haller R. and Grob P.J.
Serological investigations in 15 cases of
bird fanciers disease. Int Arch Allergy
appl Immunol 50 (1976) p. 341-358.

290. Wiseman R.D., Yoodin W.G., Miller
H.C. and Myers M.A.
Insect allergy as a possible cause of
inhalant sensitivity. J Allergy 30 (1959)
p. 191-197.

291. Chua Y.Y., Bremner K., Llobet J.L.,
Kokubu H.L., and Collins-Williams C.
Diagnosis of food allergy by the
radioallergosorbent test. J Allergy Clin
Immunol 58 (1976) p. 477-482.

292. Chua Y.Y., Bremner K., Lakdawalla N., Llobet J.L., Kokubu H.L., Orange R.P. and Collins-Williams C.
In vivo and in vitro correlates of food allergy. J Allergy Clin Immunol 58 (1976) p. 299-307.

293. Bonifazi E., Garofalo L., Monterisi A. and Meneghini C.L.
Food allergy in atopic dermatitis: Experimental observations. Acta Derm Venereol 58 (1978) p. 349-352.

294. Sennekamp J., Lange G., Nerger K., Berdel D. and Meier-Sydow J.
Human antibodies against antigens of the sparrow, blackbird, weaver finch, canary, budgerigar, pigeon and hen using the indirect immunofluorescent technique. Clin Allergy 11 (1981) p. 375-384.

295. Tsuji M., Hayashi T., Yamamoto S., Sakata Y. and Toshida T.
IgE-type antibodies to Ascaris antigens in man. Int Arch Allergy appl Immunol 55 (1977) p. 78-81.

296. Aukrust L., Apold J., Elsayed S. and Aas K.
Crossed immunoelectrophoretic and crossed radioimmunoelectrophoretic studies employing a model allergen from codfish. Int Arch Allergy appl Imunol 57 (1978) p. 253-262.

297. Elsayed L., Titlestad K., Apold J. and Aas K.
A synthethic hexadecapeptide derived from allergen M imposing allergenic and antigenic reactivity. Scand J Immunol 12 (1980) p. 171-175.

298. Karr R.M., Wilson M.R., Anicetti V.R., Lehrer S.B., Butcher B.T. and Salvaggio J.E:
An approach to fungal antigen relationships by radioallergosorbent test inhibition. J Allergy Clin Immunol 67 (1981) p. 194-198.

299. Järvinen K.A.J., Pirilae V., Björkstén F., Keskinen H., Lehtinen M., and Stubb S.
Unsuitability of bakery work for a person with atopy: A study of 234 bakery workers. Ann Allergy 42 (1979) p. 192-195.

300. Patterson R., Roberts M., Ghory A.C. and Greenberg P.A.
IgE antibody against Aspergillus fumigatus antigen i n patients with allergic bronchopulmoanry aspergillosis. Clin Exp Immunol 42 (1980) p. 395-398.

301. Patterson R., Rosenberg M. and Roberts M.
Evidence that Aspergillus fumigatus growing in the airway of man can be a potent stimulus of specific and non-specific IgE formation. Am J Med 63 (1977) p. 257-262.

302. Baldo B.A. and Wrigley C.W.
IgE antibodies to wheat flour components. Studies with sera from subjects with bakers' asthma or coeliac condition. Clin Allergy 8 (1978) p. 109-124.

303. Björksten F., Backman A., Järvinen K.A.J., Lehti H., Savilahti E., Syvänen P. and Kärkkäinen T.
Immunoglobulin E specific to wheat and rye flour proteins. Clin Allergy 7 (1977) p. 473-483.

304. Baur X.
Studies on the specificity of human IgE-antibodies to the plant proteases papain and bromelain. Clin Allergy 9 (1979) p. 451-457.

305. Kozak P.P. Jr., Gallup J., Cummins L.H. and Gillman S.A.
Currently available methods for home mold surveys. II. Examples of problem homes surveyed. Ann Allergy 45 (1980) p. 85-89.

306. Jarisch R., Roth A., Boltz A. and Sandor I.
Diagnosis of penicillin allergy by means of Phadebas RAST penicilloyl G and V and skin tests. Clin Allergy 11 (1981) p. 155-160.

307. Data on file G55. Comparison of uptake for boxer, Alsatian and poodle.

308–326 References

308. *Bruynzeel P.L.B. and Houben L.A.M.J.*
Evaluation of total and specific IgE
determinations in normal children
and children suffering from asthmatic
bronchitis with suspected allergic
disease. Clin Chim Acta 112 (1981)
p. 315-323.

309. *Barnetson R.S.C., Merrett T.G.
and Ferguson A.*
Studies on hyperimmunoglobulinaemia
E in atopic diseases with particular
reference to food allergens. Clin Exp
Immunol 46 (1981) p. 54-60.

310. *Kersten W. and Hoek G.T.*
Schimmelpilzallergie. Wien Med
Wochenschr 130 (1980) p. 275-282.

311. *Aas K., Leegaard J., Aukrust L.
and Grimmer O.E.*
Immediate type hypersensitivity to
common moulds. Comparison of
different diagnostic materials. Allergy 35
(1980) p. 443-451.

312. *Kraft D., Roth A., Mischer P., Pichler H.
and Ebner H.*
Specific and total serum IgE
measurements in the diagnosis of
penicillin allergy. A long term follow-up
study. Clin Allergy 7 (1977) p. 21-28.

313. *Sneller M.R. and Roby R.R.*
Incidence of fungal spores at the homes
of allergic patients in an agricultural
community. I. 12-month study in and
out of doors. Ann Allergy 43 (1979)
p. 225-228.

314. *Triebig G., Thürauf J., Zober A. and
Weltle D.*
Arbeitsplatzbezogener Inhalationstest
(AIT), Acetylcholintest (ACH-T) und
RAST als Beurteilungskriterien einer
berufsbedingten obstruktiven Atem-
wegserkrankung durch Mehlstaub.
Arbeitsmed Sozialmed Präventiv-
med 14 (1979) p. 232-235.

315. *Gravesen S.*
Fungi as a cause of allergic disease.
Allergy 34 (1979) p. 135-154.

316. *Perkkioe M.*
Immunohistochemical study of
intestinal biopsies from children with
atopic eczema due to food allergy.
Allergy 35 (1980) p. 573-580.

317. Data on file G55. Sensitivity to lecitin in
soy bean.

318. *Buckley R.*
Food allergy. JAMA 248 (1982) p. 2629.

319. *Gravesen S.*
Identification and prevalence of
culturable mesophilic microfungi in
house dust from 100 Danish homes.
Allergy 33 (1978) p. 268-272.

320. *Basomba A., Villalmanzo I.G., Campos
A., Pelaez A. and Berglund A.*
IgE antibodies against penicillin as
determined by Phadebas RAST®. Clin
Allergy 9 (1979) p. 515-525.

321. *Gronemeyer W.*
Über Schimmelpilzallergie.
Therapiewoche 27 (1977) p. 4339-
4350.

322. *Prince H.E. and Meyer G.H.*
An up-to-date look at mold allergy. Ann
Allergy 37 (1976) p. 18-25.

323. *Aukrust L.*
Crossed radioimmunoelectrophoretic
studies of distinct allergens in two
extract of *Cladosporium herbarum*. Int
Arch Allergy appl Immunol 58 (1979)
p. 375-390.

324. *Aukrust L. and Borch S.M.*
Partial purification and characterization
of two *Cladosporium herbarum*
allergens. Int Arch Allergy appl Immunol
60 (1979) p. 68-79.

325. *Levine M.I. and Lockey R.F.*
Eds.: Monograph on insect allergy.
Amer. Acad. Allergy Comm. on Insect.
Pittsburgh, Pa. 1981.

326. *Aukrust L.*
Cladosporium herbarum allergens. Arb
Paul Ehrlich Inst Georg Speyer Haus
Ferdinand Blum Inst 73 (1978)
p. 56-64.

327. Data on file G55. Comparison, specificity and cross-reactivity between yeast and mould

328. Virchow C., Roth A., Debelić M. and Möller E.
Radio-Allergo-Sorbent-Test (RAST) bei Schimmelpilzsporensensibilisierung. Prax Pneumol 29 (1975) p. 555-568.

329. Shibasaki M., Suzuki S., Nemoto H. and Kuroume T.
Allergenicity and lymphocyte-stimulating property of rice protein. J Allergy Clin Immunol 64 (1979) p. 259-265.

330. Rubenstein L.
Sensitivity to sesame seed and sesame oil. NY State J Med 50 (1950) p. 343.

331. Uvitsky I.H.
Sensitivity to sesame seed. J Allergy 22 (1956) p. 377.

332. Torsney P.J.
Hypersensitivity to sesame seed. J Allergy 35 (1964) p. 514.

333. Malish D., Glovsky M.M., Hoffman D.R., Ghekiere L., and Hawkins J.M.
Anaphylaxis after sesame seed ingestion. J Allergy Clin Immunol 67 (1981) p. 35-38.

334. Weiss N., Stürchler D. and Dietrich F.M.
Radioallergosorbent and indirect fluorescent antibody tests in immuno diagnosis of schistosomiasis. Lancet (1978:2) p. 1231-1233.

335. Sarsfield J.K., Boyle A.G., Rowell E.M. and Moriarty S.C.
Pet sensitivities in asthmatic children. Arch Dis Child 51 (1976) p. 186-189.

336. Enders B., Shaker Z. and Zwisler O.
Serum IgE levels in individuals infected with Schistosoma mansoni and Schistosoma haematobium. Z Tropenmed Parasitol 25 (1974) p. 75-77.

337. Berrens L.
Epidermal allergens. Rev Allergy 24 (1970) p. 917-925.

338. Brown H.W.
Basic clinical parasitology, Appleton-Century Crofts. New York 1975, p. 201.

339. Voorhorst R. and Spieksma F.
Recent progress in the house dust mite problem. Acta Allergol 24 (1969) p. 115-123.

340. Data on file G55. Comparison of onion allergens.

341. Moroz L.A. and Yang W.H.
Kunitz soybean trypsin inhibitor. A specific allergen in food anaphylaxis. NEJM 302 (1980) p. 1126-1128.

342. Ramirez D.A.
The natural history of mountain cedar pollinosis. I Allergy Clin Immunol Jan. 1984, p. 88-93.

343. Hannuksela M. and Lahti A.
Immediate reactions to fruits and vegetable. Contact Derm 3 (1977) p. 79-84.

344. Gillespie D.N., Nakajima S. and Gleich G.
Detection of allergy to nuts by the radioallergosorbent test. J Clin Allergy Immunol 57 (1976) p. 302-309.

345. Osváth P., Muranyi L., Endre L. and Harsanyi G.
Investigation of the cross reaction of cow's hair and milk antigen in bronchial provocation. Acta Allergol 27 (1972) p. 355-363.

346. Wüthrich B. and Much T.H.
Nahrungsmittel-Allergen-Testung bei Acne vularis. Dermatologica 157 (1978) p. 292-295.

347. Gravesen S., Løwenstein H. and Weeke B.
Demonstration, isolation and identification of culturable mircofungi and bacteria in horse and hair and dandruff. Immunochemical comparison with allergenic components. Allergy 33 (1978) p. 89-92.

348. Data on file G55. Sensitivity and cross-reactivity of allergen disc w17.

349. Bøg-Hansen T.C., Prahl P. and Løwenstein H.
A set of analytical electrophoresis experiments to predict the results of affinity chromatographic separations; fractionation of allergens from cow's hair and dander. J Immunol Meth 22 (1978) p. 293-307.

350. Monoret-Vautrin D.A.
In the Mast Cell. Its role in health and disease. Eds. J Pepys and A.M. Edwards. Proc. Int. Symp., Davos, Switzerland. Pitman Medical Publishing Co., Ltd. England. p. 436.

351. Prahl P., Weeke B. and Løwenstein H.
Quantitative immunoelectrophoretic analysis of extract from cow hair and dander. Characterization of the antigens and identification of the allergens. Allergy 33 (1978) p. 241-253.

352. Data on file G55. Comparison, sensitivity and specificiy of allergen discs f41, f3, m2 and g5.

353. Osváth P., Endre L. and Péter F.
Beweisführung der möglichkeit einer immunologischen Kreuzreaktion awischen Kuhmilch and Rindehaar anhand allergenspezifischer IgE-Untersuchungen. Allerg Immunol (Leipzig) 25 (1979) p. 203-206.

354. Data on file G55. Comparison, sensitivity and cross-reactivity of allergen discs f44, g5 and m2.

355. Data on file G55. Sensitivity, specificity and cross-reactivity of allergen discs f25 and f33.

356. Bousquet J., Ménardo J.L., Aznar R., Robinet-Lévy M., Michel F-B.
Clinical and immunologic survey in beekeepers in relation to their sensitization. J All Clin Immunol 73 (1984) p. 332-340.

357. Bock A.S., Lee W-Y., Remigio L.K. and May C.D.
Studies of hypersensitivity reactions to foods in infants and children. J Allergy Clin Immunol 62 (1978) p. 327-334.

358. Zulkfifli A. and Kwai Weng Chen
Experience with skin reactions to various allergens in bronchial asthma. Med J Malaysia 34 (1979) p. 153-155.

359. Bock S.A.
The natural history of food sensitivity. J Allergy Clin Immunol 69 (1982:2) p. 173-177.

360. Data on file G55. Testing for specificity and cross-reactivity of allergen disc w16.

361. Speer F.
Multiple food allergy. Ann Allergy 34 (1975) p. 71-76.

362. Data on file G55. Sensitivity, specificity and cross-reactivity of allergen discs w14.

363. Data on file G55. Sensitivity, specificity and cross-reactivity of allergen disc f37.

364. Data on file G125. Evaluation of Johnson grass and Bahia grass discs, Louisiana, USA.

365. Kang S.
13 cases of food allergy. Korean J Int Med 15 (1973) p. 23-24.

366. Wüthrich von B.
Nahrungsmittelallergie. Allergologie 4 (1981) p. 320-328.

367. Werner M.
Krankheiten infolge peroraler Allergen-invasion (Allergischer Manifestationen der Verdauungsorgane). In. Lehrbuch der klinischen Allergi, p. 179, hrsg.v.K. Hansen u. M. Werner, Thieme, Stuttgart 1967.

368. Grant E.C.G.
Food allergies and migraine. Lancet 1 (1979) p. 966-968.

369. Lahti A. and Hannuksela M.
Hypersensitivity to apple and carrot can be reliably detected with fresh material. Allergy 33 (1978) p. 143-146.

370. Read N.W., Krejs G.J., Read C.A., SantaOna C.A., Morawski S.G. and Fordtran J.S.
Chronic diarrhoea of unknown origin.. Gastroent 78 (1980) p. 264-271.

371. Aalberse R.C., Koshte V. and Clemens J.G.J. Immunoglobulin E antibodies that crossreact with vegetable foods, pollens, and Hymenoptera venom. J Allergy Clin Immunol 68 (1981) p. 356-364.

372. Data on file G55. Specificity and cross-reactivity of allergen f35.

373. Prahl P. Isolation of allergens from cow hair and dander. Allergy 35 (1980) p. 208-209.

374. Much T., Wüthrich B. and Töndury T. Zur Klinik, Diagnose und Therapie der Nahrungsmittelallergie. Z Hautkr 53 (1978) p. 141-149.

375. Prahl P. Allergens in cow hair and dander. Origin of cow allergens in the environment. Allergy 36 (1981) p. 561-571.

376. Prahl P. and Nexoe E. Human serum IgE against two major allergens from cow hair and dander. Determination of affinity and quantity of antigen-specific IgE. Allergy 37 (1982) p. 49-54.

377. MacKechnie H.L.N. The clinical spectrum of yeast hypersensitivity. Ann Allergy 39 (1978) p. 334-338.

378. Malley A., Baecher L., Mackler B. and Perlman F. Isolation of allergens from the green pea. J Allergy Clin Immunol 56 (1975) p. 282-290.

379. James J. and Warin R.P. An assessment of the role of Candida albicans and food yeasts in chronic urticaria. Br Med J 84 (1971) p. 227-237.

380. Hoffman D.R., Day E.D. and Miller J.S. The major heat stable allergen of shrimp. Ann Allergy 47 (1981) p. 17-22.

381. Burgess J.F. Occupational dermatitis due to onion and garlic. CMAJ. 66 (1952) p. 275.

382. Burks N. and Reod-Petersen J. Occupational protein contact dermatitis in food handlers. Contact Dermatitis 2 (1976) p. 28.

383. Singh S.M., Pasricha J.S., Sharma R.C. and Kandhari K.C. Vegetables responsible for contact dermatitis of the hands. Arch Dermatol 113 (1977) p. 776.

384. Ketel van W.G. and de Haan P. Occupational eczema from garlic and onion. Contact Dermatitis 4 (1978) p. 53.

385. Wüthrich B. and Arrendal H. RAST in the diagnosis of hypersensitivity to dog and cat allergens. A comparison of different extract preparations with clinical history, skin test and provocation tests. Clin Allergy 9 (1979) p. 191-200.

386. Apold J., Havnen J., Hvatum M., Oseid S. and Aas K. The radioallergosorbent test (RAST) in the diagnosis of reaginic allergy. A comparison between provocation tests, skin tests and RAST employing allergosorbents which were arbitrarily prepared with commercial allergen extracts. Clin Allergy 4 (1974) p. 401-409.

387. Berg T.L.O. and Johansson S.G.O. Allergy diagnosis with the radioallergo-sorbent test. A comparison with the results of skin and provocation tests in an unselected group of children with asthma and hay fever. J Allergy Clin Immunol 54 (1974) p. 209-221.

388. Data on file G55. Comparison of cross-reactivity and specificity of allergen discs f4, 5, 6, 7, 8, 9, 10, 11.

389. Ito K., Horiuchi Y., Kumagai M., Ueda M., Nakamura R., Kawanishi N. and Kasai Y. Evaluation of RAST as an immunologi-cal method for diagnosis of multiocular Echinococcus. Clin Exp Immunol 28 (1977) p. 407-412.

390. *Kleinhans D.*
Allergenspezifisches Immunoglobulin E im Serum (RAST) bei Tierepithelien-sensibilisierung. Med Welt 28 (1977) p. 630-633.

391. *Kleinhans D.*
Die Bedeutung des Radio-Allergo-Sorbens-Test (RAST) in der Allergiediagnostik. Therapiewoche 29 (1979) p. 3608-3622.

392. *Ohman J.L., Lowell F.C. and Bloch K.J.*
Allergens of mammalian origin: Characterization of allergen extracted from cat pelts. J Allergy Clin Immunol 52 (1973) p. 231-241.

393. *Brandt R., Ponterius G. and Yman L.*
The allergens of cat epithelia and cat serum. Comparative studies based on the radioallergosorbent technique (RAST). Int Arch Allergy 45 (1973) p. 447-455.

394. *Ohman J.L., Lowell F.C. and Bloch K.J.*
Allergens of mammalian origin. III. Properties of a major feline allergen. J Immunol 113 (1974) p. 1667-1668.

395. *Özkaragoez K., Smith H.J., Gökçen M. and Saraçlar Y.*
The radioallergosorbent test (RAST) in the diagnosis of atopic allergy. Acta Allergol 29 (1974) p. 96-100.

396. *Rudolph R., Meier-Duis H., Kunkel G., Staud R.D. and Stock U.*
Über die Bedeutung von Tierhaar-allergien bei Erkrankungen der oberen Luftwege. Dtsch Med Wochenschr 100 (1975) p. 2557-2561.

397. *Brehm K., Plock K., Doepp M. and Baier H.*
Antigenität des Serumalbumins bei Allergie gegen Katzen- und Hundeepithelien und Bedeutung des Radioallergosorbents-Tests in der Allergiediagnostik. Dtsch Med Wochenschr 100 (1975) p. 472-476.

398. *Stokes C.R. and Turner M.W.*
Isolation and characterization of cat allergens. Clin Allergy 5 (1975) p. 241-254.

399. *O'Donnell I.J. and Mitchell G. F.*
An investigation of the allergens of *Ascaris lumbricoides* using a radioallergosorbent test (RAST) and sera of naturally infected humans: Comparison with an allergen for mice identified by a passive cutaneous anaphylaxis test. Aust J Biol Sci 31 (1978) p. 459-487.

400. Data on file G55. Testing for mould sensitivity among nut-sensitive patients.

401. *Ohman J.L. Jr., Bloch K.J., Kendall S. and Lowell F.C.*
Allergens of mammalian origin. IV: Evidence for common allergens in cat and dog serum. J Allergy Clin Immunol 57 (1976) p. 560-568.

402. *Ohman J.L. Jr., Lowell F.C., Bloch K.J. and Kendall S.*
Allergens of mammalian origin. V. Properties of extracts derived from the domestic cat. Clin Allergy 6 (1976) p. 419-428.

403. *Løwenstein H.*
Characterization and chemical modification of isolated allergens from horse hair and dandruff. Int Arch Allergy appl Immunol 57 (1978) p. 349-357.

404. *Koers W.J., Young E. and Berrens L.*
Animal dander allergy. Clin Allergy 7 (1977) p. 245-253.

405. *Ohman J.L. Jr., Kendall S. and Lowell F.C.*
IgE antibody to cat allergens in an allergic population. J Allergy Clin Immunol 60 (1977) p. 317-232.

406. *Merrett J. and Merrett T.G.*
RAST atopy screen. Clin Allergy 8 (1978) p. 235-240.

407. *Merrett T.G. and Merrett J.*
Epithelial or dandruff allergen for the diagnosis of dog allergy by RAST? Clin Allergy 9 (1979) p. 429-435.

408. *Brandt R. and Yman L.*
Dog dander allergens. Specificity studies based on the Radioallergo-sorbent technique. Int Arch Allergy appl Immunol 61 (1980) p. 361-370.

409. *Hoffman D.R.*
Dog and cat allergens: Urinary proteins or dander proteins? Ann Allergy 45 (1980) p. 205-206.

410. *Guerin B. and Jewott B.*
A comparative study of allergen extracts from cat fur, cat pelt and cat saliva. Ann Allergy 46 (1981) p. 127-131.

411. *Anderson M.C. and Baer H.*
Allergenically active components of cat allergen extracts. J Immunol 127 (1981) p. 972-975.

412. *Schultze-Werninghaus G.*
Atemwegserkrankungen durch Soforttypallergie gegen Tierepithelien. Allergologie 4 (1981) p. 298-303.

413. *Brighton W.D., Topping M.D. and Berry J.B.*
Allergene aus Katzenfell. Allergologie 4 (1981) p. 270-275.

414. *Debelić M. and Bahmer F.*
Die bedeutung von RAST in der Diagnostik der Tierhaarallergie. Allergologie 4 (1981) p. 249-255.

415. *Løwenstein H.*
Allergene von Katze, Hund, Rind und Pferd. Allergologie 4 (1981) p. 265-269.

416. *Ohman J.L. Jr., Marsh D.G. and Goldman M.*
Antibody responses following immunotherapy with cat pelt extract. J Allergy Clin Immunol 69 (1982) p. 319-326.

417. *Staud von R.D., Rudolph R., Baumgarten C., Kunkel G. and Sladek M.*
Immunoglobulinverläufe von gesamt- und spezifischen IgE bei Tierhaar-Allergikern nach Tierhaar-karenz. Allergologie 5 (1982) p. 75-80.

418. *Markussen B., Løwenstein H. and Weeke B.*
Allergen extract of horse hair and dandruff. Quantitative immuno-electrophoretic characterization of the antigens. Int Arch Allergy appl Immunol 51 (1976) p. 25-37.

419. *Blands J., Løwenstein H. and Weeke B.*
Characterization of extract of dog hair and dandruff from six different dog breeds by quantitative immuno-electrophoresis. Identification of allergens by crossed radioimmuno-electrophoresis (CRIE). Acta Allergol 32 (1977) p. 147-169.

420. *Holford-Strevens V.*
Allergenic activity of cat and dog skin fractions obtained by Sephadex gel filtration. Clin Allergy 3 (1973) p. 225-234.

421. *Løwenstein H., Markussen B. and Weeke B.*
Isolation and partial characterization of three major allergens of horse hair and dandruff. Int Arch Allergy appl Immunol 51 (1976) p. 48-67.

422. *Yman L., Brandt R. and Ponterius G.*
Serum albumin – an important allergen in dog epithelia extracts. Int Arch Allergy 44 (1973) p. 358-368.

423. *Løwenstein H., Markussen B. and Weeke B.*
Identification of allergens in extract of horse hair and dandruff by means of crossed radioimmunoelectrophoresis. Int Arch Allergy appl Immunol 51 (1976) p. 38-47.

424. *Varga J.M. and Ceska M.*
Characterization of allergen extracts by polyacrylamide gel isoelectrofocusing and radioimmunosorbent allergen assay. II. Dog and cat allergen. Int Arch Allergy 42 (1972) p. 438-453.

425. *Aronsson T. and Wide L.*
Studies on allergens of horse epithelium with two variants of RAST. Int Arch Allergy 47 (1974) p. 224-241.

426. *Ponterius G., Brandt R., Hulten E. and Yman L.*
Comparative studies on the allergens of horse dandruff and horse serum. Int Arch Allergy 44 (1973) p. 679-691.

427. *Weeke B.*
Fractionation and purification of allergens from dogs and cats. In: Adv Allergol appl Immunology. Proc Xth Int Congr of Allergol. Jerusalem 1979. Ed. by E Oehling. Oxford and New York (Pergamon Press) 1980. p. 499-504.

428. *Yman L., Blomberg F. and Schröder H.*
Characterization of dog and cat allergens. Direct specific detection of electrophoretically separated allergens by means of IgE antibodies and enzyme anti-IgE. In: Adv in Allergology and Immunology. Proc Xth Int Congr of Allergol. Jerusalem 1979. Ed by A Öhling. Oxford and New York (Pergamon Press) 1980. p. 499-504.

429. *Leegaard J. and Roth A.*
RAST in the diagnosis of hypersensitivity to horse allergens. Clin Allergy 7 (1977) p. 455-464.

430. *Pécoud A., Ochsner M., Arrendal H. and Frei P.C.*
Improvement of the radioallergosorbent test (RAST) sensitivity by using an antibody specific for the determinant $D_\varepsilon 2$. Clin Allergy 12 (1982) p. 75-81.

431. *Moore B.S. and Hyde J.S.*
Breed-specific dog hypersensitivity in humans. J Allergy Clin Immunol 66 (1980) p. 198-203.

432. *Brown H.M., Thantrey N., Su S. and Jackson F.A.*
Rassenspezifische allergie gegenüber Hunden. Allergologie 4 (1981) p. 256-260.

433. *Fagerberg E. and Wide L.*
Diagnosis of hypersensitivity to dog epithelium in patients with asthma bronchiale. Int Arch Allergy appl Immunol 39 (1970) p. 301-309.

434. Data on file G 118. De Filippi I. and Hoffman R. Evaluation of laboratory prototypes of corn and soybean RAST discs.

435. *Rudolph R., Kunkel G., Blohm B., Muckleman R., Mast H., Kirchhof E. and Sladek M.*
Zur haeufigheit und klinischen Bedeutung von allergien gegen Tierepithelien. Allergologie 4 (1981) p. 230-231.

436. Data on file G55. Comparison, sensitivity and cross-reactivity of allergen discs t16, t3, g5 and m2.

437. *Haahtela T. and Jokela H.*
Asthma and allergy in Finnish conscripts. Allergy 34 (1979) p. 413-420.

438. *Holopainen E., Salo O.P., Tarkiainen E. and Malmberg H.*
The most important allergens in allergic rhinitis. Acta Otolaryngol (1979): Suppl. 360, p. 16-18.

439. Data on file G55. Research report. Comparison of *Quercus robur* and *Quercus alba*.

440. *Hoffman D.R. and Shipman W.H.*
Allergens in bee venom. I. Separation and identification of the major allergens. J Allergy Clin Immunol 58 (1976) p. 551-562.

441. Data on file G55. Research report. Comparison of cross-reactivity among different *Ulmus* species.

442. Data on file G55. Sensitivity and cross-reactivity of t14 compared to t12, t3, g5 and m2.

443. *Wüthrich B. and Kopper E.*
Bedeutung des Radio-Allergo-Sorbens-Test (RAST) in der spezifischen Diagnostik des atopischen Asthma bronchiale. Dtsch Med Wochenschr 103 (1978) p. 603-609.

444. *Ceska M., Eriksson R. and Varga J.M.*
Radioimmunosorbent assay of allergens. J Allergy Clin Immunol 49 (1972) p. 1-9.

Index

We have included the common names for grass, weed and tree pollens and animals in English, French, Italian, German, Spanish and Dutch to help you find the correct plant. The Latin is given here and in the text. A separate list of the Japanese plants follows this index.

A

Index

Index

Index

Index

Index

Index

Index

Index

アレルゲン

G1	ハルガヤ		W13	オナモミ
G2	ギョウギシバ		W14	アオゲイトウ
G3	カモガヤ		W16	ニワトコ
G4	ヒロハノウシノケグサ		W18	ヒメスイバ
G5	ホソムギ		W20	イラクサ
G6	オオアワガエリ		T1	トネリコバカエデ
G7	ヨシ		T2	ハンノキ
G8	ナガハグサ		T3	シラカンバ
G9	コヌカグサ		T4	ムラサキハシバミ
G10	ヒメモロコシ		T5	ブナノキ
G11	コスズメノチャヒキ		T6	ヤマノビャクシン
G13	ビロードグサ		T7	オーク
G16	スズメノテッポウ		T8	アメリカニレ
G17	スズメノヒエ		T9	オリーブ
G70	ライグラス		T10	クルミノキ
G71	クサヨシ		T11	スズカケノキ
W1	ブタクサ		T12	ヤナギ
W2	セイヨウブタクサ		T13	ヒロハハコヤナギ
W3	オオブタクサ		T15	アメリカトネリコ
W4	ニセブタクサ		T16	マツ
W5	ニガヨモギ		T17	ニホンスギ
W6	ヨモギ		T18	ユーカリ
W7	ノギク		T19	アカシア
W8	タンポポ		T20	メスキート
W9	ヘラオオバコ		T21	カユプテ
W10	シロアカザ		T22	ヒッコリー
W11	オカヒジキ		T23	イタリアイトスギ
W12	アキノキリンソウ		T70	クワノキ